FACE SECR

GREGORY LANDSMAN

The Beauty Advisor to Supermodels

Published by:
Wilkinson Publishing Pty Ltd
ACN 006 042 173
Level 4, 2 Collins St Melbourne,
Victoria, Australia 3000
Ph: +61 3 9654 5446
www.wilkinsonpublishing.com

International distribution by Pineapple Media Limited
(www.pineapple-media.com) ISSN 2203-2789

Design: Spike Creative www.spikecreative.com.au

Photos and Illustrations by agreement with GL SKINFIT INSTITUTE.

National Library of Australia Cataloguing-in-Publication entry

Creator: Landsman, Gregory, 1963- author.

Title: Face secrets / Gregory Landsman.

ISBN: 9781925265576 (paperback)

Subjects: Face – Care and hygiene.
            Skin – Care and hygiene.

Dewey Number: 646.726

I have always felt that my purpose in life was to share a message about the truth of
beauty; that it is a God given right for all to experience it if they are willing to embrace,
celebrate and accept not only their differences, but the differences in our world. The truest
embodiments of this are often children and animals, who are both perfect reflections of
living fully without awareness or concern for their physicality, or the comparisons that
inevitably ensue from that. My passion to support both our children and our animals
stems not only from a deep compassion for the true beauty they represent, but similarly
their vulnerability in this world. They act as powerful reminders that we need to be
mindful in the way we live and love ourselves and others; including the animals that
bring so much love and beauty to this world. All of my author royalties from this book
will be donated. Proceeds will be provided to two primary causes – supporting cranio-
facial reconstructive surgery for children, and saving animals in need of support. At the
moment our focus is on elephants. I believe that when we feel compassion, we are moved
inwardly and our hearts reach out to the needs of others. In this state we access the belief
that we all have the ability to contribute to making our world a more beautiful place;
whether that is simply practicing acceptance of peoples differences or sharing a kind
word or deed.

'As individuals we can make a change, together we can make a difference.'

Gregory Landsman

FACE SECRETS IS A NATURAL ANTI-AGEING PHENOMENON THAT WILL SHOW YOU HOW TO COUNTERACT THE DAY TO DAY STRESS & TOXINS THAT AGE YOUR SKIN.

With the right approach we can retain and maintain healthy glowing skin, counteract deep wrinkles and maintain skin firmness and health at any age. This is what I call being 'SKINFIT'.

HOW WE AGE IS 100% CONTROLLABLE ON A DAILY BASIS!

In my 30 years working with faces and skin in the beauty industry I have had the opportunity to work with some of the world's largest names in fashion and beauty; collaborate with world class chemists to develop ground breaking skin products; provide advice to supermodels on their skin health; and speak with thousands of women and men of all ages on skin and the ongoing challenge to look as good as we can for as long as we can.

As a result I have concluded that there are three essential things that can be done to support the skin to maintain its strength, vitality and youthful glow:

1. Remove the impacts of stress from the skin on a very regular basis
2. Deeply hydrate the skin
3. Feed it the right skin building vitamins and minerals

Each of these steps is about DE-STRESSING the skin and restoring its natural health.

When we de-stress our skin, we naturally age less!

These are the principles and foundation of the face lifting formulas I developed for models to keep their skin fresh and glowing, and now use to develop products to support Practitioners.

They are also the principles that underpin each of the DIY steps in this book.

Each of the formulas in *Face Secrets* feature ingredients that are acknowledged by science as some of the most powerful skin 'anti-agers' available today and are designed to target our greatest skin concerns, such as reducing fine lines and wrinkles, improving firmness and elasticity and protecting our skin from free radicals that cause premature ageing.

So the good news is that it doesn't matter how old you are, whether you're a supermodel, super woman, or super mother, the powerful anti-ageing secrets in this book can support you to de-stress and provide you with the keys to look younger, feel younger and stay younger.

WHAT REALLY AGES THE SKIN...

Daily stress as well as poor diet, lack of sleep and unhappy thoughts play havoc with our faces, profoundly affecting the way our skin and bodies visibly age.

Yet from my experience and approach to beauty, looking younger is actually much easier than we have been led to believe.

With the right approach we can retain and maintain healthy glowing skin, counteract deep wrinkles and maintain skin firmness and health at any age. In other words, 'GET SKINFIT'!

From the overwhelming response to my previous books, I have been inspired to create *Face Secrets*, a compilation of some of the most powerful formulas and insights that can help you look younger, feel younger and stay younger.

Face Secrets takes you on a journey and arms you with the knowledge and power to reclaim your own brand of beauty, starting with your face and ending with your heart.

The first key to getting SKINFIT is to de-stress your skin, giving it a break from stress and everyday toxins.

We all know that life in general can be stressful and as a result our skin carries enormous amounts of stress, not only from the environmental toxins we are exposed to but daily stress of every kind.

And then there is of course the stress of ageing, the anxiety of noticing the first grey hair, or being smacked in the face by your first wrinkle.

Regardless of what kind of stress is in our lives, the first place it shows up is on our faces.

In this book I will share the approach I have shown to people of all ages wanting to achieve younger looking skin and deal with what they often consider to be their skin challenges: dry skin, fine lines and wrinkles, and sagging or dull looking skin.

However, the first thing I tell them is that the secret to improving your skin is dealing with stress and the impact it has on our skin, as well as the toxins that we are exposed to on a day to day basis through the foods we eat, which will also have an effect on our bodies and our skin.

But that isn't the whole story. A large part of seeing our beauty and feeling it is understanding that there is an indelible link between the way we look and the way we feel.

Through my years in the fashion and beauty industry and my personal experiences I have always believed in many ways that women become more beautiful as they age. I saw this with my mother and grandmother, women from every country, and the models I worked with. I have also seen it in my wife of 21 years.

Somehow, women seem to develop a self confidence and a stronger presence that was not evident in their youth.

So while their physical appearance shows a life well lived, what makes them truly beautiful is how they wear their lines and the way they feel about themselves and their lives. I firmly believe that this brand of beauty has no expiry date and is genuinely ageless. Beauty is not exclusive to models and movie stars and certain physical characteristics. It is inclusive of every woman and her individuality.

While *Face Secrets* is about nurturing your face and your body to get SKINFIT, it is also about knowing that the beauty we find outside ourselves is a very small aspect of what lies within.

While I have seen supermodels in Paris dressed in Chanel and women in India dressed in rags, the one truth that reveals their beauty, regardless of who they are, is the truth of their smile.

Our journey to discover the truth about beauty is a personal one that we all make, but if we solely use our eyes to see our beauty, we will only see limited aspects of what makes us beautiful.

So whether you are indulging in a skin rejuvenating bath or giving yourself a three-minute facial, reclaiming the fullness of your beauty is an adventure worth embarking on. After all, BEAUTY is about good living and great loving; it is about feeling more, healing more, living more and loving more.

Stay blessed and beautiful.

Gregory Landsman

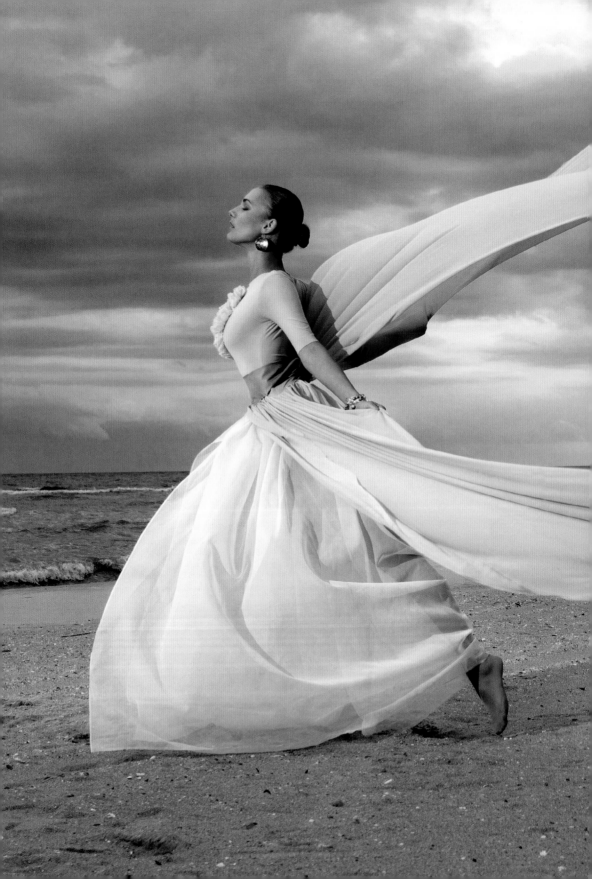

LET ME GROW GRACEFULLY
LET ME AGE GRATEFULLY

LET ME DO THIS
Beautifully
— GREGORY LANDSMAN

A MESSAGE FOR THE READER

While all treatments in this book are skin-friendly, everyone has unique skin that reacts differently. It is recommended with all treatments that a patch test be performed on a small non-sensitive area of skin (such as your hand) prior to using. If redness, a rash or any form of irritation occurs, wash off immediately and discontinue use.

No information contained in this book is to be used as medical advice and *Face Secrets* is not to be used to diagnose, treat, cure or prevent any medical condition. Before relying on the following information, you should carefully evaluate the accuracy and relevance of the material for their purposes and obtain appropriate professional medical advice. You must consult a qualified medical professional if you have any questions regarding any skin condition or concerns.

Please note that the ingredients listed are used as a guide only, so feel free to adjust treatments according to your own needs and sensitivities.

As a general rule, ensure that your work area and utensils are clean before preparing any treatments or recipes, and that ingredients are fresh and your hands are washed. This will support the freshness and quality of each treatment.

Please note that treatments that contain Alpha Hydroxy Acid (AHA) and Retinol (vitamin A) can cause the skin to be sun sensitive, so always apply sun protection to any area where these treatments have been used.

CONTENTS

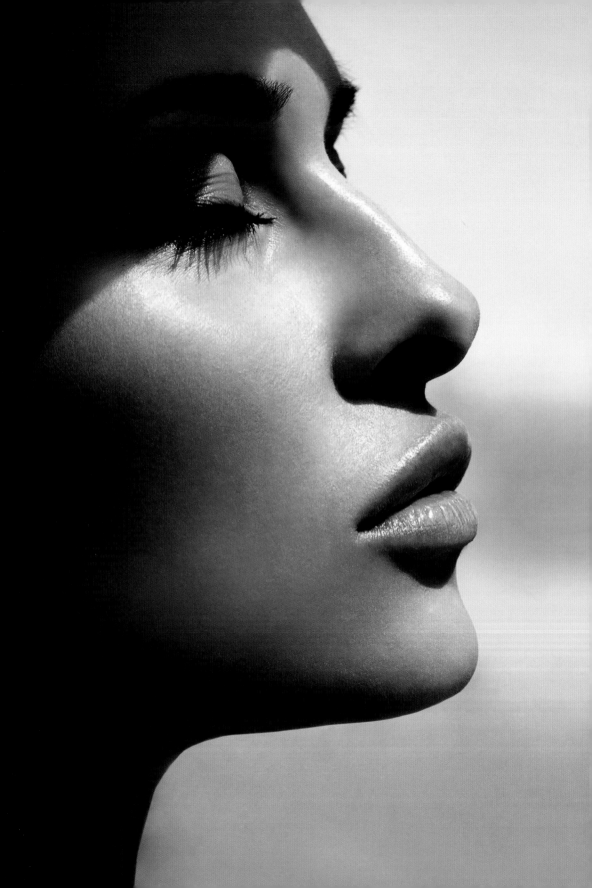

DE-STRESS YOUR SKIN & AGE LESS!

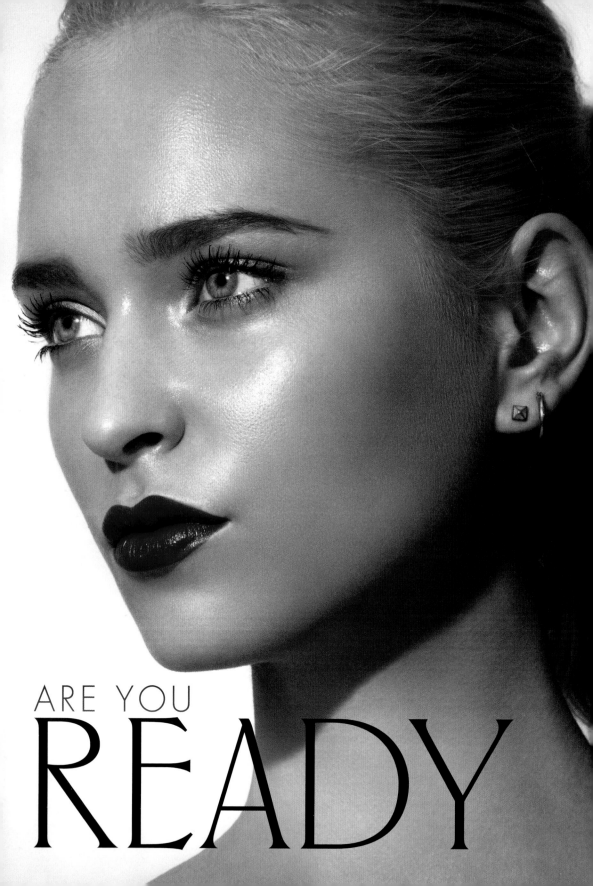

ARE YOU
READY

TO
LOOK
YOUNGER
FEEL
YOUNGER
AND
STAY
YOUNGER?

To get

SKINFIT

We need to deal with one of the
biggest culprits that ages our skin

STRESS!

STRESS IN OUR WORLD IS AT AN ALL TIME HIGH!

Living in the modern day world generally comes with a whole lot of stress! Whether that means coping with a high pressure job; juggling home and work; raising a family; maintaining relationships; or trying to get enough rest and 'me' time ... many of us are often stretched to the limit.

We generally assume stress only impacts our mental or emotional state, and yet the truth is that stress is one of the greatest 'ageing' factors for our skin. Why? Because it depletes the body of essential vitamins and minerals, impacting cell repair and production of connective tissue, **accelerating the ageing process.**

Most people's skin is suffering from
stress
overload

STRESS + SUN + EVERYDAY TOXINS + POLLUTION ALL AGE THE SKIN!

We live in a world where stress has become the 'norm' and our everyday lives expose us to toxins of many kinds.

Exposure to UV rays; eating food that isn't 100% homemade; pollution; air conditioning and heating (just for starters) all have an impact on the skin.

So we are now at a point where the world in which we live exposes us to stress and toxins on a daily basis. Yet in reality there is no escaping this. That is, unless you are prepared to give up your favourite makeup, move to a pollution free country and eat only the food you grow yourself, while never being exposed to UV rays. Hardly a practical solution for most!

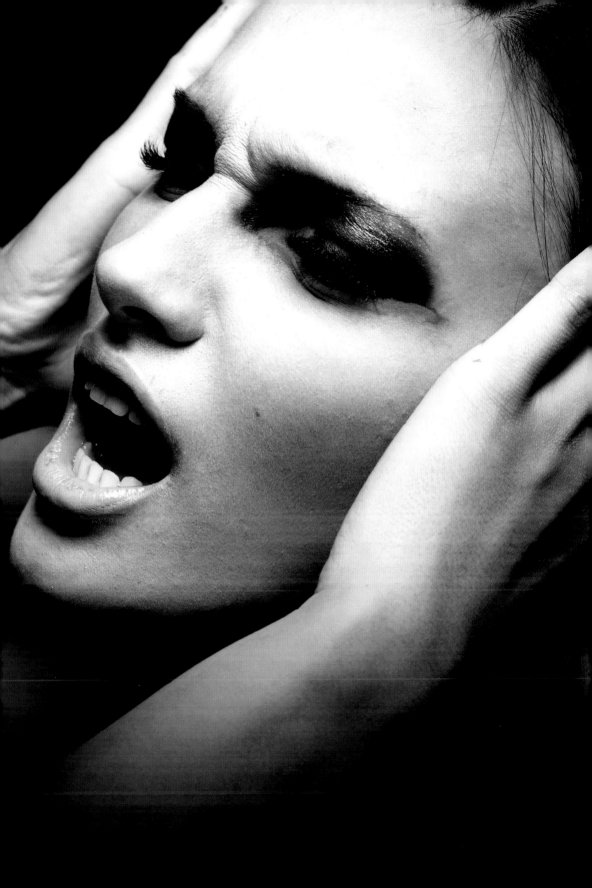

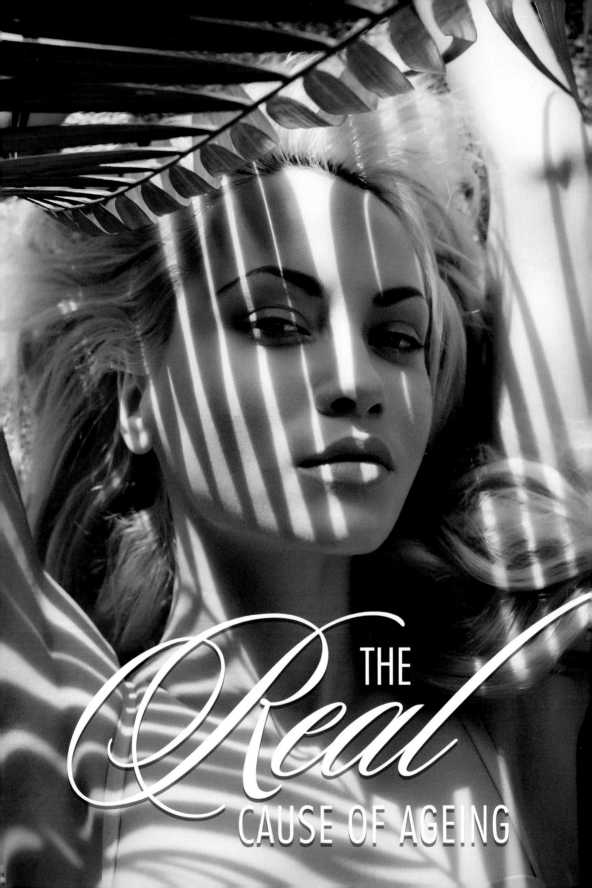

THE *Real*
CAUSE OF AGEING

The stress hormone called 'cortisol' is one of three hormones released by the adrenal glands into the blood stream when we are under any form of stress.

Now I don't know a person who has a stress free life, as stress has become an unavoidable part of modern day living. The foods we eat, the number of hours we sleep, and the quality of our sleep all contribute to our stress levels, which can add years to your face and accelerate the ageing process.

This wouldn't be a problem if this only occurred every now and then, but research shows that most of us are now living with what has been termed 'chronic stress', or stress that doesn't allow the hormones that support us when we are combating stress to recede back to normal.

The *stress* hormone that causes
Wrinkles

Experts tell us that we are suffering from a state known as 'chronic stress', or stress that just never goes away.

As a result we are in a constant state of stress and worry and our faces and bodies are suffering the impact of this.

STRESS HORMONES AGE THE FACE AND CREATE WRINKLES

When we are feeling stressed the adrenal glands release cortisol. When this happens, sugar levels in the blood naturally increase, and the increased blood sugar promotes 'glycation' in our skin and damages our collagen.

Cortisol also decreases our skins' natural production of hyaluronic acid, which acts as a natural moisturiser for our skin. On top of this it compromises the skin's barrier, which allows even more hydration to be lost; and when skin is dehydrated, the enzymes in our skin that work to repair the damage don't work as well.

CORTISOL ISN'T THE ONLY BY-PRODUCT OF STRESS THAT IMPACTS THE SKIN

Adrenaline brought on by stress also works against our complexions. When adrenaline is present, blood flow to the skin is decreased, which robs it of vital nutrients, including oxygen. Less oxygen and sluggish circulation in general leads to a dull, sallow complexion.

The long term impact of daily stress can be seen on our skin and shows up on faces causing us to look and feel older than we are. After all, worry lines are just that, evidence of too much cortisol from stress that sits on the face!

The good news is that we can counteract stress, giving our skin the opportunity to renew and revive and as we do so we will not only reduce fine lines, but over time we will naturally 'wrinkle less'. My motto is that when we de-stress we age less!

WE NEED TO destress

OUR SKIN SO WE AGE LESS

Skin building vitamins and minerals are typically found in fruits, vegetables and grains.

To give your skin the very best opportunity to look fresh, and stay fresh looking, we need to find a way to deliver vitamins and minerals to the skin on a regular basis, thereby reducing the impact of toxins from makeup and the environment.

With that in mind this book features recipes that will build the skin and bring the glow back. I have also included a series of my own recommendations for ongoing maintenance, including stress relief and the supplements that are essential for skin health.

WHY vitamins & minerals?

Medical peak bodies and academic institutions the world over acknowledge that toxins, lack of sleep and stress contribute meaningfully to premature ageing of the skin and that prevention is supported by ingesting vitamins and minerals that feed the body and the skin.

The Dermatological industry has confirmed that using vitamins directly onto the skin can make a significant difference to maintaining younger looking skin, more so than merely taking vitamin tablets.

Vitamins are essentially antioxidants that work to neutralise oxidative damage from toxins within the deeper skin layers. This is best achieved transdermally, through topical application directly on the impacted skin. So while vitamins work to counter the damage from toxins and stress, skin-building minerals are important for strengthening the connective tissue essential for healthy collagen and elastin.

Experts agree that if you wear makeup every day you need to feed your skin vitamins and minerals!

So to give our skin the best chance of staying strong and healthy, we need to counteract what is depleted by stress and toxins. This means that anyone who wears makeup every day needs to give their skin a break and feed it the vitamins and minerals that can balance the day-to-day stresses that age the skin.

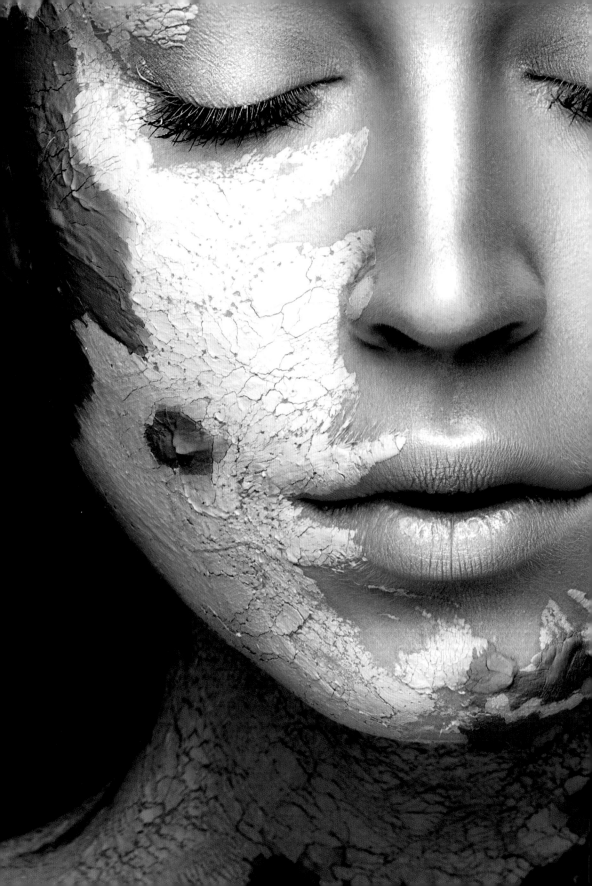

THE POWER OF A GREAT
mask

Our skin is an incredible self-maintaining organ.

It never ceases to amaze me that every 28 days it renews itself and provides us with fresh new cells, revealing radiant new skin. However as we age, this process slows down and can leave the skin looking uneven and dry, which leads to fine lines and premature ageing. At this point it is essential to give your skin some support.

Masks are vastly underrated as an anti-ageing approach and are a powerful weapon in the fight against stress-induced skin damage. The three biological functions in masks essential to help de-stress the skin work in a very short time.

A good mask:

1. Removes dead skin cells, cleanses pores and smooths and improves texture while reducing fine lines.

2. Aids the skin in boosting circulation and retaining optimal moisture levels.

3. Delivers vitamins, minerals and antioxidants to help strengthen the skin.

Of course not every mask will do this, but those worth their 'salt' will deliver a kick-start to your de-stress, age less beauty routine. A good mask delivers great results for younger looking skin.

The optimal use of a mask is weekly. That way you ensure that what is sitting on your skin from the week is removed and you set your skin up to absorb further nutrients and healing from other products.

The treatments on the following pages will help kick-start the skin de-stress process.

TIGHT, BRIGHT AND BEAUTIFUL skin renewing FACE PACKS

DIY face packs not only cleanse the skin, they also maintain the tautness while removing waste from pores that have been inundated with chemicals, environmental pollutants, oil, dirt impurities and dead skin cells.

Some face packs you can make easily and use in minutes, making them one of the easiest ways to counteract toxins and stress.

Regardless of your age it is time to shine. So whether you are heading to work, staying at home or getting ready for that special occasion, there is no reason that your skin shouldn't say, 'I am vital, healthy and radiant!'

These face packs help your skin say it loud and clear.

Cucumber skin renewal face pack for oily skin

You will need:

- 1 tablespoon cucumber juice
- 1 tablespoon lemon juice
- ½ teaspoon peppermint extract

How to make it:

1. Mix all the ingredients together and apply to the face.

2. Leave on for twenty minutes.

3. Wash off with lukewarm water.

THE GL SKINFIT SECRET THAT DELIVERS REAL RESULTS

This treatment cleanses, purifies and detoxifies skin while renewing it with powerful antioxidants, vitamins A and C, trace minerals and enzymes essential for skin growth and repair.

FILL YOUR EYES
WITH SMILING
CLOUDS, LISTEN
TO THE BIRDS
AND CELEBRATE
THE BODY THAT
CONTINUALLY
ALLOWS YOU
TO TASTE THE
GOODNESS AND
RICHNESS OF

Life

IT IS TIME
TO AWAKEN
TO THE

Beauty

WE ALL
POSSESS
AS HUMAN
BEINGS, TO
EMBRACE AND
EXPERIENCE
OURSELVES IN
A LOVING AND
FULFILLING WAY

- GREGORY LANDSMAN

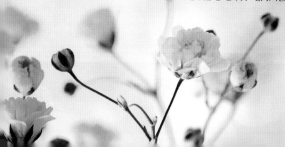

PEEL AND REVEAL

radiant fresh NEW SKIN

Masks and peels are left on for a specific length of time, increasing the amount of active ingredients that penetrate the skin. With peels, the degree to which the bonds between dead skin cells break apart and disappear is determined in part by how long you allow the acids to work. It's best to use peels sparingly. The biggest mistake women make is applying peels daily as this can overstress the skin. Peels can contribute to sun sensitivity too.

Green apple face mask

You will need:

- 1 green apple
- 2 teaspoons loose leaf chamomile tea (or 1 teabag)
- 2 teaspoons loose leaf green tea (or 1 teabag)
- 1 package of unflavoured gelatin
- 1 tablespoon fresh orange juice

How to make it:

1. Remove the seeds from the apple and blend the flesh to a pulp in a food processor. Strain the solids through a piece of gauze and keep the juice for later.

2. Boil some water and make ½ cup (125ml) of chamomile tea and ½ cup (125ml) of green tea. Let the tea stand for a few minutes and then strain until you have ¼ cup (60ml) of each.

3. Add the gelatin, chamomile and green teas to a small pan. Gently warm the mixture up over a low heat while constantly stirring, until the gelatin is completely dissolved. Add the cucumber and tomato juices and the aloe vera gel and mix well. Let the mixture cool down and place the bowl in the fridge until it is firm and almost set but still liquid enough to be applied, about 25–30 minutes.

4. Stir the mixture to see if it is the right thick consistency, if so spread the paste gently and equally with a facial mask brush or spatula on your clean face and neck, making sure to keep the eye and upper lip area clear.

5. Leave the mask on until it dries, about 20–30 minutes.

6. Once dry, gently peel the mask off, start under your chin and peel it off in an upward motion, this will tingle a bit. Finally rinse your face with warm water and apply moisturiser onto damp skin.

GL SKINFIT
Secret

This facial peel nourishes and revitalises.

Green apples are amazing for the skin and are rich in vitamins A, C and B6, and minerals iron, zinc and calcium. They contain a high percentage of vitamin C, which makes them potent antioxidants, and have better skin polishing ingredients than regular apples. Tired and stressed out skin breathes in new life with this treatment. The malic acid in the apples is a powerful exfoliator that removes dead skin cells. Chamomile and green teas soothe and alleviate puffiness and nourish and moisturise the skin. Orange juice is rich in citric acid, which gently removes dead skin cells while boosting the skin with vitamin C. This treatment also helps restore collagen in your body, which is responsible for skin firming and prevents premature ageing of the skin. Oranges contain powerful antioxidants that fight the free radicals often responsible for wrinkles and sagging.

sweeten up YOUR SKIN

Strawberries and honey face mask

You will need:

- 1 tablespoon dark organic honey
- ¼ cup fresh strawberries
- ¼ cup fresh sour grapes
- 1 teaspoon fresh lemon juice
- 2 tablespoons plain unflavoured yoghurt

How to make it:

1. Warm up the honey until it becomes runny but not hot. To do this, place the honey in a small glass or metal bowl immersed in hot water.

2. Place the strawberries and grapes in a food processor and mash them to a pulp.

3. Add the honey, lemon juice and yoghurt and mix until a smooth paste forms.

4. Spread the paste gently and equally with a spatula or face mask brush on your clean face and neck, making sure to keep the eye area clear.

5. Lie down, relax and leave the mask on for 15 minutes.

6. Wash the mask off with lukewarm water and end with a splash of cold water. Pat your skin dry with a clean towel.

THE GL SKINFIT SECRET THAT DELIVERS REAL RESULTS

This treatment uses natural acids to exfoliate your skin. The yoghurt contains lactic acid that gently exfoliates the skin. Strawberries are rich in Salicylic acid and aid in beautifying skin by removing impurities and dead skin cells that accumulate on the surface, giving it a healthy glow. The vitamin C and zinc content in strawberries strengthens the skin and supports the production of collagen, reducing fine lines and wrinkles.

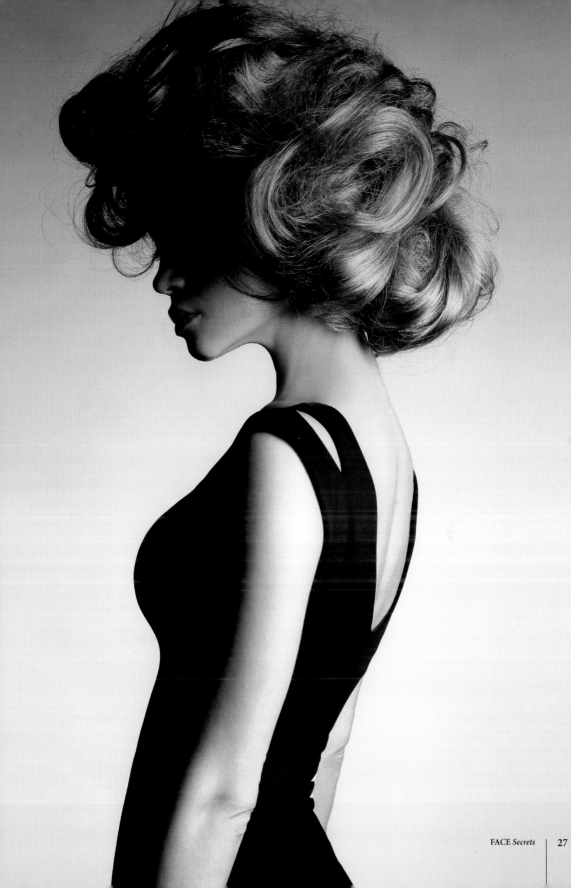

EGG IT ON FOR A

brighter tighter COMPLEXION

Our skin is the mirror of our lifestyle. As we go through our day, driving, working, meeting deadlines, dealing with traffic jams and last minute shopping, daily stresses can all play havoc on our skin and finding the time for pampering can be difficult. So when time is our most precious commodity, it makes sense to save it.

This treatment is a great time and skin saver and a great excuse to make quiet time to relax and pamper yourself.

Egg mask

You will need:

- 1 egg for a two-day treatment that you can do on a weekend

How to make it:

1. Separate the egg yolk from the white.

2. Put the egg white in a bowl and cover. Use the yolk first.

3. Beat the yolk and use a pastry brush to apply it (thickly) to a clean face and neck.

4. Leave this treatment on for 20 minutes to dry and let your skin soak up the goodness. This mask will beautify your skin and works towards hydrating and changing the quality and texture of your skin. When it dries it feels strange on the skin and it looks even stranger, but it will give you a good laugh and I think laughter has an enormous amount of skin benefits (often more than anything you can find in a jar, as it flushes your face with vitality, relieves stress and keeps you young at heart!).

5. Rinse the egg off in cool water.

6. The egg yolk is moisturising but removes impurities, leaving your skin looking naturally healthy. Apply moisturiser afterwards and feel the difference.

7. The next day use the egg white in the same way. This mask helps tighten and refine the skin and pores. Once the egg white is dry, rinse it off with cool water and apply moisturiser while your skin is damp. This will lock the moisture in.

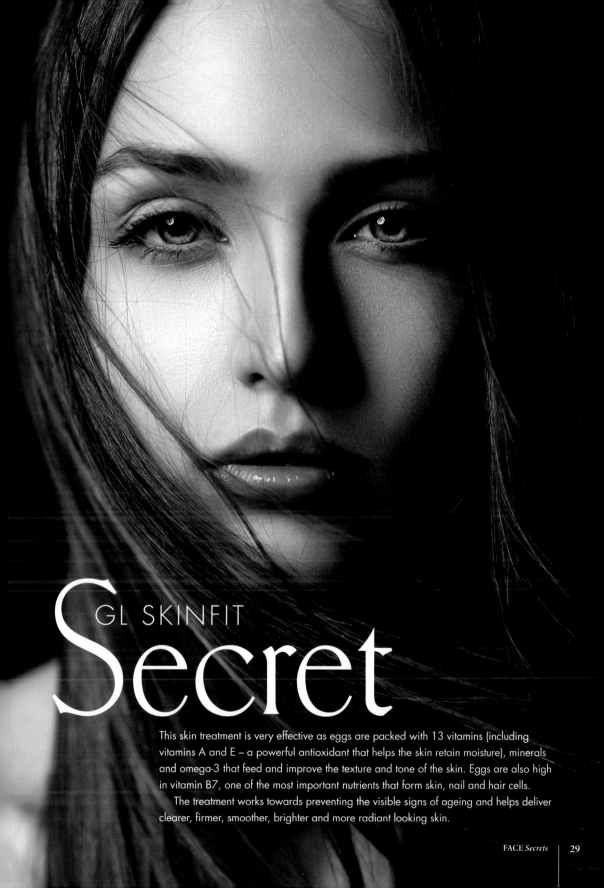

GL SKINFIT
Secret

This skin treatment is very effective as eggs are packed with 13 vitamins (including vitamins A and E – a powerful antioxidant that helps the skin retain moisture), minerals and omega-3 that feed and improve the texture and tone of the skin. Eggs are also high in vitamin B7, one of the most important nutrients that form skin, nail and hair cells.

The treatment works towards preventing the visible signs of ageing and helps deliver clearer, firmer, smoother, brighter and more radiant looking skin.

Whether the source of our stress is the endless challenge of trying to balance work and family; re-evaluating purpose once children have grown; or just no down time to smell the roses, it is important that we recognise when we are suffering from stress overload.

Here are some thoughts on how to manage the overload.

1. Regularly check in with yourself to ask whether you are nurturing yourself and your needs for a bit of balance. Everyone needs a bit of 'me' time and some nurturing.

2. When you are feeling overwhelmed by what is on your plate, ask for help!

3. Remember some of the things you loved to do most as a child (getting on a swing, playing cards etc) and go and do some of them.

4. Start a journal to record your thoughts, feelings and dreams, as they are often a great road map to help us know which road we need to take.

5. Look closely at your beliefs about who you are and what it means for you to get older. Find role models that will support you to challenge any outdated and limiting beliefs about age and beauty.

6. Let go of worrying what others think of you and focus on how you think about yourself. (Make sure you are not suffering from the 'disease to please others' at the expense of your own happiness!)

ARE YOU DEALING WITH *stress*

Working with women I see so many stress triggers in their lives that create emotional and physical wear and tear.

7. Acknowledge every day that you are part of the miracle of life and at the end of each day spend a couple of minutes being grateful for who you are. (The secret to having a positive outlook is seeing the beauty in the small things in life, such as the simple act of breathing or the smell of coffee or fresh bread first thing in the morning.)

8. Slow down, breathe deeply and ask yourself regularly: are you living the life you know you deserve? If not, find ways to retrieve abandoned dreams and plans.

9. Practice not judging others, as this can be reflective of the harsh judgments we place on ourselves.

10. When you feel upset give yourself permission to do it openly and honestly. Everyone feels better after a good cry!

11. Ensure you are getting enough serotonin, either with a capsule, some very gentle early morning sun, or eating a diet rich in vitamin D foods, such as salmon, mackerel and tuna. Vitamin D is a key player in supporting and increasing the serotonin levels in our brain. Serotonin is a chemical that helps reduce stress and anxiety and supports us to feel good.

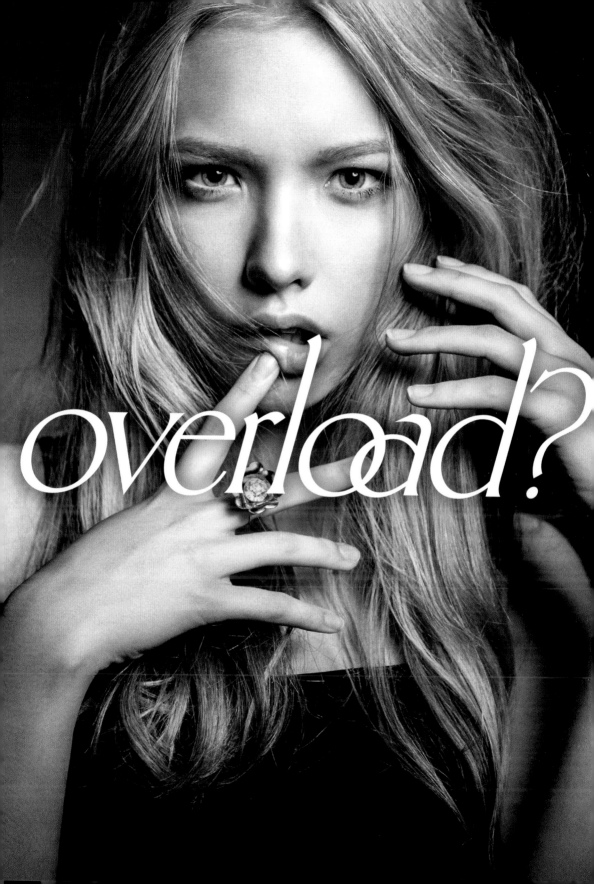

destress

YOUR SKIN BY LEARNING TO CONTROL THE STRESS HORMONE CORTISOL

Eat cortisol-lowering foods to de-stress and power up your collagen.

What you eat makes a difference not only to your health but how calm you feel and how well you cope with stress.

Protein in the diet can help reduce cortisol production and are often a good source of vitamins and minerals, which supports the overall health of skin. These include fish, eggs, meat, poultry, dairy and foods such as soybeans, rice, pea, hemp and vegetable proteins.

Healthy fats

Omega-3 fatty acids are vital for skin health but can also lower cortisol levels. Fish oil is known to lower cortisol levels and increase serotonin in the brain.

Omega-3 can also be found in flaxseed oil and canola oil. Other good fat sources include avocados, nuts and seeds, olive oil and egg yolks.

- Goji berries
- Walnuts
- Sesame seeds
- Pumpkin seeds
- Soybean oil
- Salmon
- Mackerel
- Sardines
- Anchovies
- Dark green lettuce
- Brazil nuts
- Sunflower oil
- Sesame oil

Foods rich in vitamin C

Vitamin C reduces the secretion of cortisol.

Good sources of vitamin C include:
- Sweet red pepper
- Broccoli
- Strawberries
- Papaya
- Lemon (and other citrus fruits)
- Brussels sprouts
- Cantaloupe
- Tomato
- Cucumber

Vitamin B Complex

Vitamin B Complex has a variety of B vitamins that are great for the skin and is used by the body when it is under stress.

Good sources of group B vitamins include:
- All lean red meats
- Fish
- Chicken
- Turkey
- Eggs
- Organ meats (kidney, liver)
- Prawns
- Pork
- Milk (and other dairy products)
- Almonds
- Seeds
- Beans
- Green leafy vegetables
- Carrots
- Turnips
- Celery
- Rice bran
- Soy

Foods rich in magnesium

Magnesium reduces cortisol levels and is a muscle relaxant.

Good sources of magnesium include:
- Salmon
- Soybeans
- Brown rice
- Almonds
- Avocado
- Banana
- Green vegetables
- Spinach
- Milk
- Yoghurt
- Oatmeal

Low-glycaemic carbohydrates

Low-glycaemic carbohydrates can also support the body to lower cortisol levels naturally. Make sure to avoid sugary carbohydrates that can lead to insulin surges, which cause body fat storage.

Lower glycaemic foods include:
- Brown rice
- Whole wheat bread and pasta
- Sweet potatoes
- Beans
- Vegetables

Cortisol surges after intense physical activity so be sure to eat a serve of 'good' carbohydrates immediately after you have done some exercise.

THREE MINUTE MIRACLE skin revival

FACIAL TO DE-STRESS YOUR SKIN

When there is no time for a facial and your skin is finding it hard to keep up with your hectic lifestyle, this treatment will wake up and de-stress weary skin.

This treatment is one that I formulated for women who are time poor. I always advise models to use this treatment, especially when they are travelling, on location or after a long day in front of the camera.

It is one of the easiest ways to revive tired, stressed skin and is a powerful skin and time saving treatment that fits with every lifestyle.

De-stress face mask

You will need:

- 2 teaspoons Epsom salts
- 1 tablespoon any store bought facial cleansing cream
- 1 teaspoon lemon juice
- Cool water

How to make it:

1. Wash your face with warm water.

2. Mix the Epsom Salts into the facial cleansing cream.

3. Add the lemon juice and mix together well.

4. Massage the mixture onto the skin using firm upward strokes.

5. Rinse your face with cool water.

6. Apply moisturiser to damp skin.

THE GL SKINFIT SECRET THAT DELIVERS REAL RESULTS

The alpha hydroxy acid in lemon juice renews skin cells while the magnesium in Epsom salts relaxes and de-stresses the facial muscles.

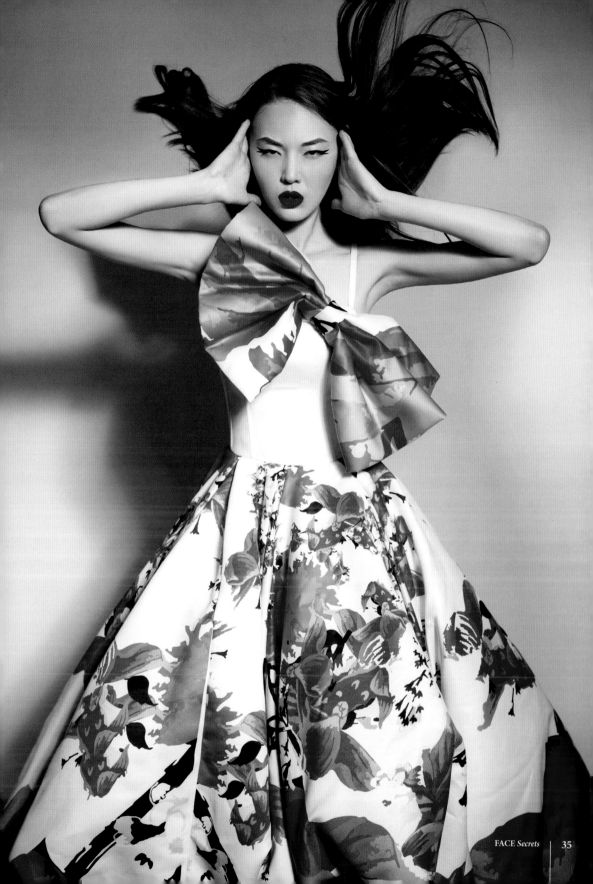

QUICK EFFECTIVE skin conditioning
FACIAL HAIR REMOVAL

This treatment moisturisers and stimulates collagen and elastin production while gently removing facial hair. It is quick to make and easy to apply.

Facial hair removal mask

You will need:

- 1 teaspoon yoghurt
- 1 tablespoon corn flour
- ½ teaspoon lemon juice

How to make it:

1. Mix the yoghurt and corn flour together.

2. Add the lemon juice and mix thoroughly until it forms a paste.

3. Apply the paste thickly all over the area where you would like to remove the hair or all over your face (avoiding the eye area) and allow it to dry.

4. To remove, rub the dried paste off in the opposite direction of the facial hair.

5. Rinse with warm water.

THE GL SKINFIT SECRET THAT DELIVERS REAL RESULTS

The yoghurt contains skin-renewing lactic acid, vitamins A and B5, and acts as a gentle exfoliant while increasing the moisture content in the skin. Lemon is a good source of alpha hydroxy acid, which removes dead skin cells. Corn flour contains the antioxidant selenium, magnesium and several B vitamins that support the moisture levels of the skin.

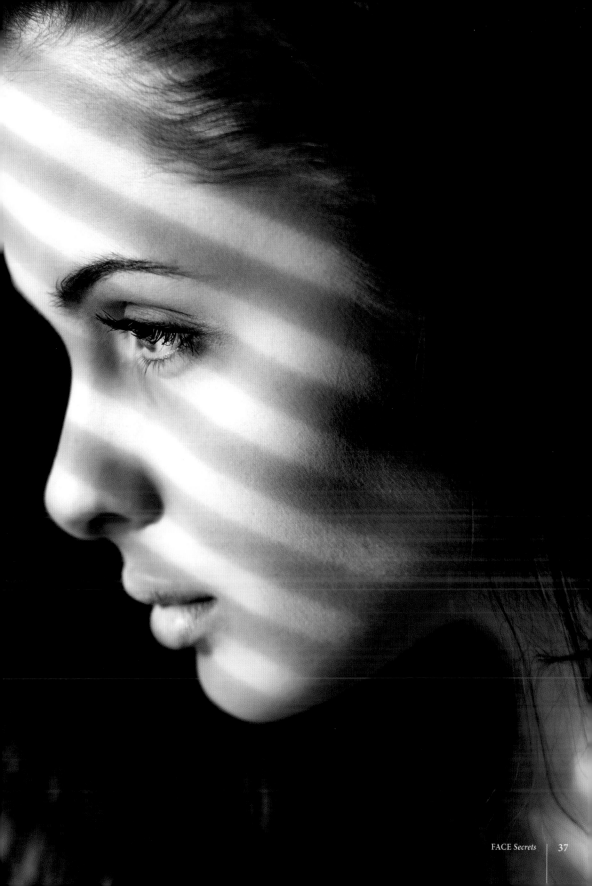

OUR **breath** IS OUR SECRET STOREHOUSE THAT HELPS US SUSTAIN CLARITY, CENTREDNESS AND A *happy* HEART

– GREGORY LANDSMAN

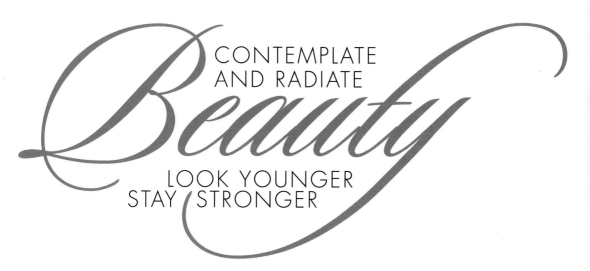

CONTEMPLATE
AND RADIATE
Beauty
LOOK YOUNGER
STAY STRONGER

There is a strong theme currently filtering through our lives as we all become more conscious of the need to make time to relax, to smell the roses, enjoy the sun and take in the fresh air.

Deep breathing is a powerful anti-ageing technique and has a direct impact on our health and our skin, while relieving stress and relaxing the body and the mind.

Whenever we make the time to enjoy these moments, we become very aware of how little time we actually take to relax and enjoy the simple things in life and the goodness they bring.

One of the unsung heroes of daily stress relief is taking 5-10 minutes to breathe deeply and consciously, as following our breath has the power to relax our body and our mind and help us manage stressful thoughts.

When we feel relaxed, our lives and the world we live in become less chaotic. We approach ourselves and the challenges in our relationships with more calmness, we feel more joyful and are capable of sharing that joy with those around us.

Through the calmness of our breath we can achieve a spiritual connection, reminding us to know our self worth and the value in living.

THE Beauty Breath

Just taking a few minutes to breathe deeply every day can make you feel better and look better.

There are several deep breathing techniques. The one that I prefer is a technique that uses the abdominal muscles.

To start, simply breathe in through your nose and breathe deeply filling your stomach up with air. The sound will remind you of gushing wind.

Hold your breath and then slowly exhale through your nose. As you are exhaling tighten the muscles of your stomach to push all air out of the lungs.

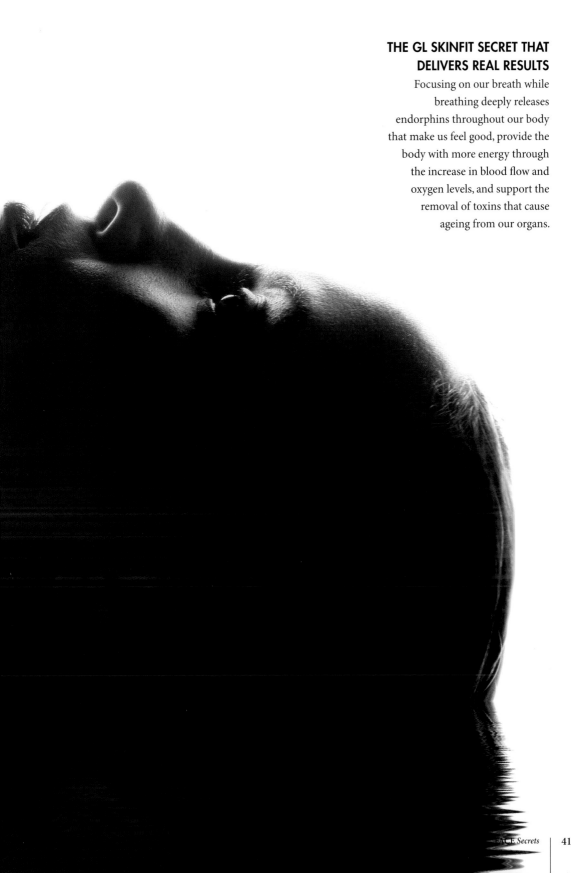

THE GL SKINFIT SECRET THAT DELIVERS REAL RESULTS

Focusing on our breath while breathing deeply releases endorphins throughout our body that make us feel good, provide the body with more energy through the increase in blood flow and oxygen levels, and support the removal of toxins that cause ageing from our organs.

A total solution TO BEAUTY

The first thing to understand is that a genuine beauty solution that lasts the test of time is not only about the creams we put on our face, and that skin health is more than just waging war on wrinkles. A youthful, healthy complexion also reflects the way we think, the way we eat, the way we live and the way we love.

Looking our best is about using what Mother Nature has given us and then focusing on our quality of life, not just the quality of our skin.

A powerful antioxidant face de-stressing mask

We are all exposed to free radicals that cause premature ageing, but the way to counteract and combat them is with powerful antioxidants.

This treatment certainly helps you do that. To help prevent premature ageing and to give skin a healthy vibrant glow, the skin's pores need to be cleansed and detoxed regularly. This supports products to be absorbed more effectively and removes chemical toxins left by cosmetics and day-to-day exposure to pollution.

You will need:

- 6 seedless grapes
- ½ teaspoon baking soda
- 1 small Lebanese cucumber
- 1 teaspoon grape seed oil

How to make it:

1. Mash the grapes up in a tea strainer to extract 1 tablespoon of grape juice. The grapes are full of alpha hydroxy acid, a powerful anti-ageing ingredient that will soften fine lines and improve skin clarity.

2. Add the baking soda. This is a gentle exfoliant that removes dead skin cells, but the real treasure is its ability to help neutralise the skin's pH balance.

3. Grate the cucumber and add to the mixture. Cucumber is rich in the mineral sulphur and promotes beautiful skin. It also contains antioxidants and skin building vitamins A, B, C and D.

4. Mix in the grape seed oil. Grape seed oil is chock-full of antioxidants and gives skin a boost of vitamins A, E and K.

5. Gently massage the mixture onto your face in small circular motions and leave it on for 20 minutes.

6. Rinse your face with warm water.

GL SKINFIT
Secret

The combination of these ingredients cleanses the skin, gently exfoliating it and leaving it smoother, while the natural infusion of antioxidants and skin brightening ingredients refresh, nourish and de-stress your skin.

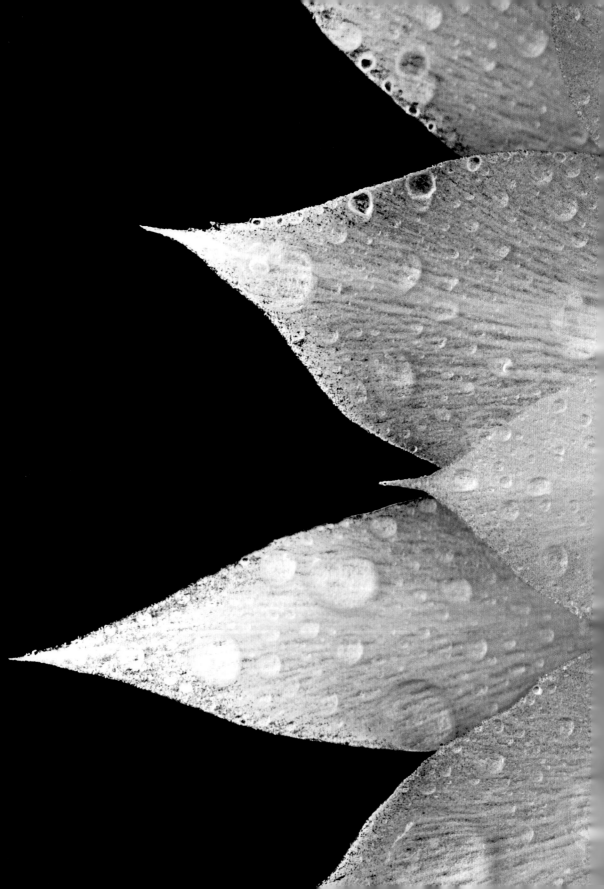

DE-STRESS, HYDRATE & PLUMP UP YOUR SKIN

The secret to younger skin is closer than you think!

WHY IS *water* IMPORTANT?

Water wonders to give you a mini detox, plump up your skin and get it glowing!

Water increases hydration, which improves the body's assimilation of food, vitamins and nutrients and improves waste elimination.

To raise our vitality we need enough water to replenish and turn over the water molecules in our bodies' cells so we don't feel sluggish and our cells are not stagnant.

When we don't have enough water our skin suffers. Ninety millilitres of water evaporate from our skin each day, so ensuring we drink a minimum of eight glasses of water daily is one of the most powerful and simple ways to hydrate our skin.

Drinking warm water is especially good for cleansing and eliminating impurities from the body and is one of the simplest ways to change your body and your skin for the better.

YOU CAN BOOST COLLAGEN AND HELP FIRM YOUR SKIN NATURALLY BY ADDING LEMON TO YOUR WATER

When it comes to keeping skin vibrant and youthful I am a BIG fan of plain water, but in saying that I love a squeeze of lemon juice in some warm water first thing in the morning.

Lemon is a vitamin C-rich citrus fruit and adding some juice to your water is one of the simplest ways to stimulate our collagen and keep our skin firm and healthy.

I have come to know that our skin responds to what is pure, so start and end the day with a mini detox for the liver.

Having recommended the lemon water ritual to supermodels, super women and super mothers all around the world, I can say with certainty that lemon water has the ability to cleanse, firm and tone our skin up. Drinking lemon water daily can make a huge difference to the appearance of your skin.

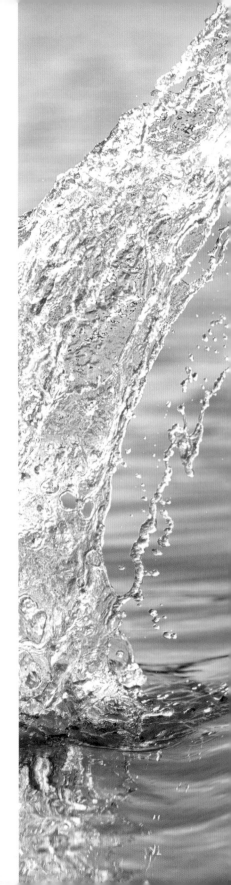

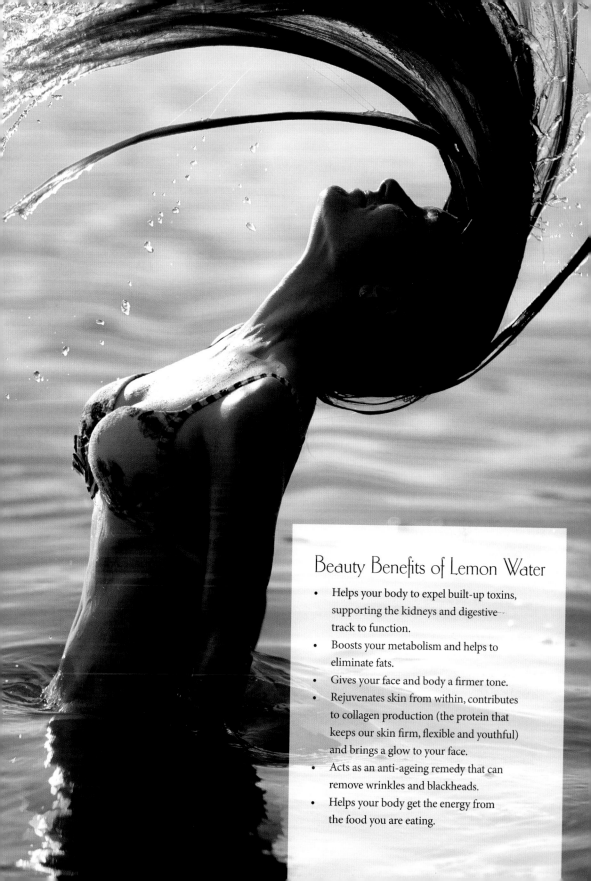

Beauty Benefits of Lemon Water

- Helps your body to expel built-up toxins, supporting the kidneys and digestive track to function.
- Boosts your metabolism and helps to eliminate fats.
- Gives your face and body a firmer tone.
- Rejuvenates skin from within, contributes to collagen production (the protein that keeps our skin firm, flexible and youthful) and brings a glow to your face.
- Acts as an anti-ageing remedy that can remove wrinkles and blackheads.
- Helps your body get the energy from the food you are eating.

FACE LIFTING FAT
plump up
YOUR
skin

Smooth out fine lines with good fats

If you are seeing fine lines appearing and your skin lacks radiance and a healthy glow, chances are you not getting enough fatty acids, and no amount of moisturiser will give that to you.

If you are serious about getting your skin and health into top gear then one of the easiest ways to take years off your skin is to ensure that you add enough essential fatty acids to your diet. This is the 'maestro moisturiser' that works from the inside out.

Our skin cell walls are made of fat and so I can always tell when a model's skin is ageing prematurely, as more often than not they are on a low fat diet! Now don't worry, despite all the low fat food marketing, good fats full of omega-3 taken in moderation won't make you fat, but they will plump up your skin and smooth out fine lines.

Low fat equals dull, dry, lacklustre skin! I always recommend including essential fatty acids in the diet and in my '5 Day Face Lifting Formula' because good fat equates to healthy, youthful looking skin.

Good fats are not to be feared but to be eaten regularly as they help your body regenerate. Fatty acids are a wrinkle-fighting weapon that will get your skin back on track.

When we do not getting enough fatty acids the cell walls cannot keep their shape, which in turn leads to dull, saggy, aged looking skin. That is why when we lose fat through fad diets our skin looks older than it is. Eating low fat, high sugar foods accelerates the process as sugar breaks down collagen, a double negative impact on your skin!

Consuming good fats is one of the most important aspects of skin care and the smartest way to plump up the skin and smooth out fine lines. And since our body does not produce essential fatty acids we must ensure we are feeding our body enough of them. They are called 'essential' because our body and the health of our skin rely on them.

GL SKINFIT Secret

These healthy fats work hard to keep our skin cells at the top of their game so they keep all the good things in, like water and nutrients, and simultaneously rid the body of waste.

Youthful skin is full of buoyant, plump, water-filled cells. But our skin cells' ability to hold water slowly decreases with age, so essential fatty acids help the cells retain water. This in turn nourishes our skin, giving it a radiant and beautiful appearance. To boost body and skin health, keep omega-3 levels topped up simply by adding them to your diet.

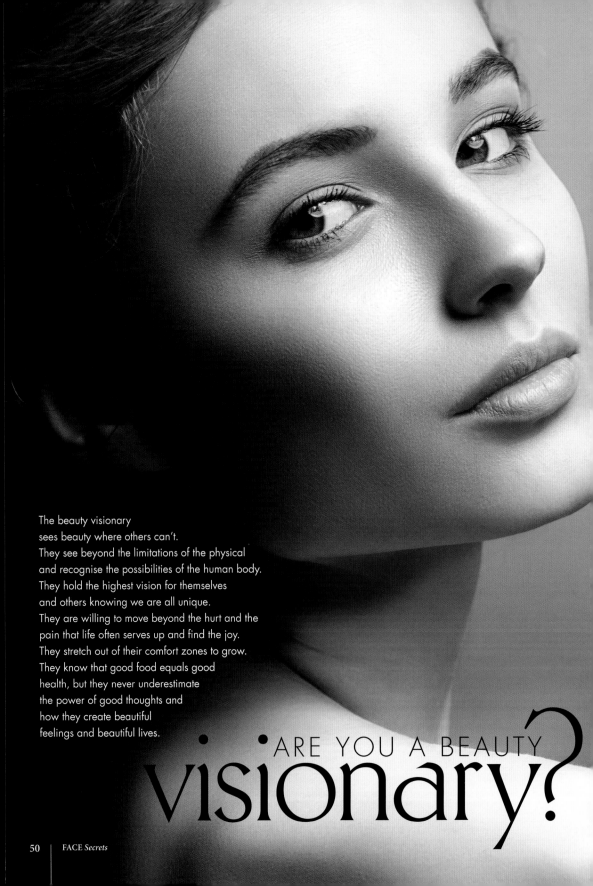

The beauty visionary
sees beauty where others can't.
They see beyond the limitations of the physical
and recognise the possibilities of the human body.
They hold the highest vision for themselves
and others knowing we are all unique.
They are willing to move beyond the hurt and the
pain that life often serves up and find the joy.
They stretch out of their comfort zones to grow.
They know that good food equals good
health, but they never underestimate
the power of good thoughts and
how they create beautiful
feelings and beautiful lives.

ARE YOU A BEAUTY
visionary?

BYE BYE puffy eyes

We all know what it is like to wake up with puffy eyes and a face that feels like it needs to be nurtured and nourished. This treatment is powerful and effective, it will help remove the swelling under the eyes.

In India basil is regarded as a herb that protects homes from evil but in this case it helps get rid of puffy eyes, which some people consider evil. It is a humble herb that has been used for thousands of years as an anti-ageing remedy. Basil is loaded with antioxidants such as flavonoids that protect you on the cellular level, and vitamins for proper organ function. This sweet smelling powerhouse packs a healthy punch for such a small ingredient.

Green tea is not only a healthful brew helping us regain our good health due to a high concentration of antioxidants, but is also an effective remedy for dark circles under the eyes. Green tea is rich in anti-inflammatory, anti-microbial and anti-irritant medicinal properties. While we know that green tea is full of antioxidants, what isn't commonly known is it contains polyphenols, specifically tannins. Polyphenols are potent enough to easily penetrate the skin's surface. The tannins in tea are astringent substances that shrink body tissues and when you apply it topically it has a tightening effect on the skin's surface.

Puffy eyes skin tightening and protecting treatment

You will need:

- 2 tablespoons fresh basil
- 2 tablespoons loose leaf organic green tea (or 1 teabag)

How to make it:

1. Boil the basil and green tea in a small pan with 1 cup (250ml) of water.

2. Wait for 5 minutes until it cools then strain the tea.

3. This potent treatment can be used on your eyes or whole face. To reduce puffiness soak cotton wool eye pads in the cooled tea, lie back and relax for 10 minutes with the pads on your eyes.

THE GL SKINFIT SECRET THAT DELIVERS REAL RESULTS

Green tea is rich in anti-inflammatories and contains powerful antioxidants but it also contains tannins that shrink body tissues and have a tightening effect on skin when applied topically.

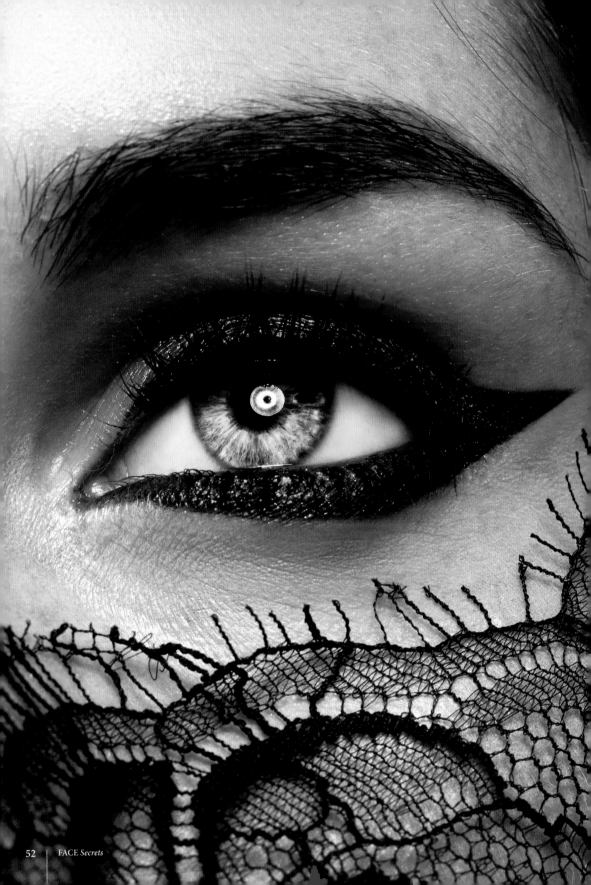

REBUILD
skin II
collagen
AND IMPROVE THE TONE AND TEXTURE OF YOUR SKIN

Skin boosting treatment

You will need:

- 2 tablespoons organic honey
- 2 medium sized carrots
- 1 egg
- ½ ripe avocado
- 2 tablespoons olive oil

How to make it:

1. If necessary warm up the honey to make it runny.

2. Steam the carrots until you can easily mash them. Add the carrots and the rest of the ingredients to a food processor and mix until you have a smooth cream.

3. Use your fingertips to smooth the paste gently and equally over your clean face and neck, making sure to keep the eye area clear.

4. Lie down, relax and leave the mask on for 15-20 minutes.

5. Wash the mask off by alternating between cold and warm water, end with a splash of warm water.

6. Apply moisturiser onto damp skin.

THE GL SKINFIT SECRET THAT DELIVERS REAL RESULTS

Avocados are rich in antioxidants and loaded with fatty acids, which work together to feed the skin, plumping it up and smoothing fine lines. The skin strengthening antioxidants in Grape seed oil hydrate the skin and protect it from premature ageing. Your skin will feel hydrated, retextured and energised. Carrots are loaded with vitamin A (in the form of beta-carotene), vitamin C, calcium, potassium, magnesium, phosphorus and various other vitamins and minerals that enhance skin tone and increase its firmness and elasticity.

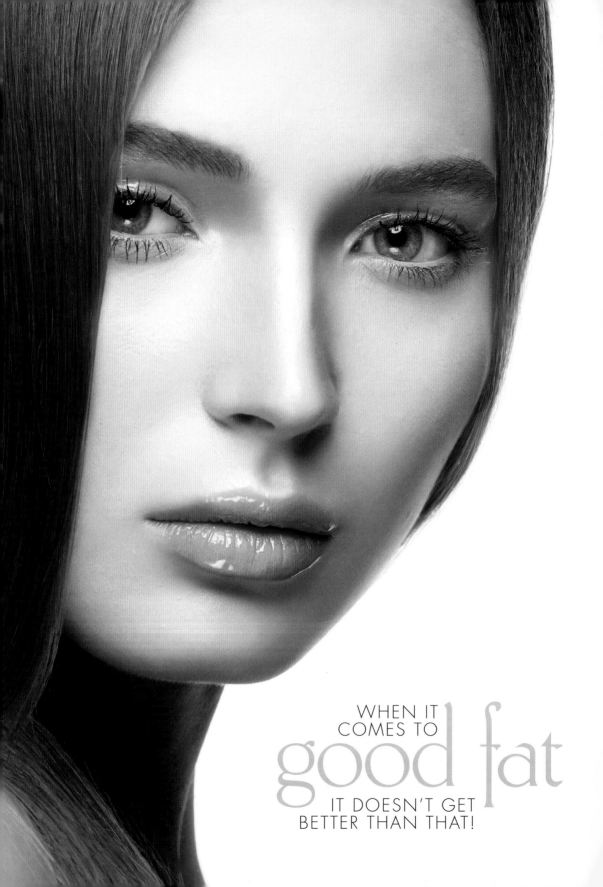

WHEN IT
COMES TO
good fat
IT DOESN'T GET
BETTER THAN THAT!

skin Beautifying

REASONS TO INCLUDE FATTY ACIDS IN YOUR DIET

1. Keeps the skin strong, healthy and flexible.
2. Makes your skin more elastic and more resistant to oxidative damage from the sun.
3. Smooths out fine lines and plumps up the skin.
4. Moisturises the skin from the inside out.
5. Hydrates cells and keeps them watertight, which firms up the skin and means less wrinkles and more skin elasticity.
6. Supports your body to absorb and move nutrients easily.
7. Helps produce the skin's natural oil barrier – critical in keeping skin hydrated, plump and younger looking.
8. Omega-3 fats have an anti-inflammatory effect that can help to calm irritated skin, giving you a clear, smooth complexion.

So the next time you are in the supermarket add a few omega-3 fatty acid ingredients to your basket that will help give you the skin results you're looking for, and start eating your way to tighter, brighter looking skin.

Omega-3 rich foods that will add radiance to your skin:

- Walnuts
- Sardines
- Salmon
- Mackerel
- Flaxseed
- Flaxseed oil
- Safflower oil
- Soy
- Fortified eggs

I have seen people achieve incredible skin results by simply adding fatty acids to their diet.

Including a few of these in your daily diet will get your skin flying in the right direction, leaving it with a youthful, radiant look as well as plumping up and smoothing out fine lines. If you have not eaten enough omega-3 rich meals lately, take a good fish oil or cod liver oil supplement to top them up.

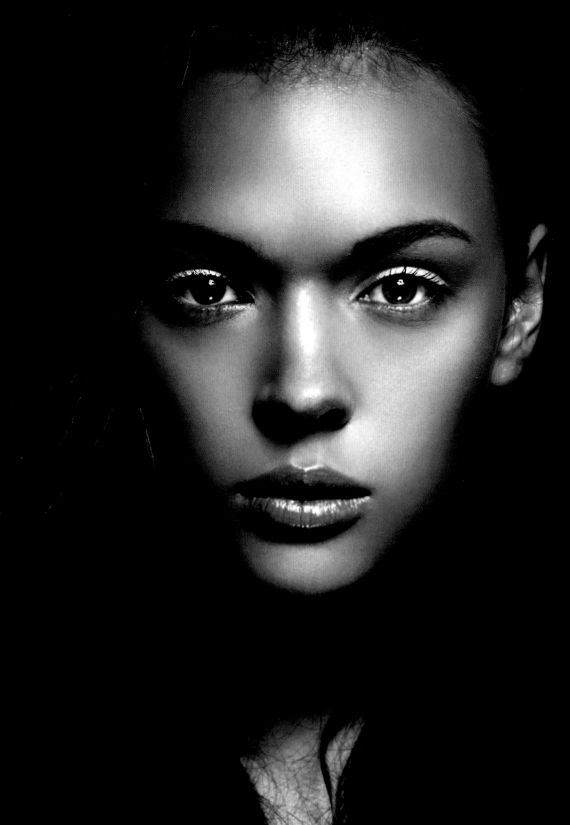

Tighten AND brighten

YOUR SKIN WITH VITAMINS AND MINERALS

Vitamin and mineral mask

You will need:

- 1 tablespoon organic honey
- 1 tablespoon rolled oats
- ½ cucumber
- 1 teaspoon plain unflavoured yoghurt
- 1 tablespoon aloe vera juice

How to make it:

1. Warm up the honey until it becomes liquid by putting it in a small glass or metal bowl that is immersed in hot water.

2. Add the oats to a blender with the cucumber, yoghurt and aloe vera juice. Blend everything well until you have a smooth paste.

3. Add the mixture to the honey.

4. Spread the paste gently and equally with a facial mask brush or spatula on your clean face and neck, making sure to keep the eye area clear.

5. Lie down, relax and leave the mask on for 20 minutes.

6. Wash the mask off with lukewarm water then apply a moisturiser to your damp face, this way you seal your skin to keep the moisture inside.

THE GL SKINFIT SECRET THAT DELIVERS REAL RESULTS

Oats are loaded with saponins, which are natural cleansers. They are full of lubricating fats that prevent dull skin and support the skin's natural barrier function, leaving it radiant. Honey is a natural humectant that holds water in the skin for maximum moisture and gives skin a healthy glow. The aloe vera juice is full of amino acids, skin boosting vitamins and minerals to soothe inflamed skin and enhance collagen, and hyaluronic acid to help rejuvenate skin. Aloe vera juice is packed with skin boosting vitamins A, C, E, B1, B2, B3, B6, B12 and folic acid. It's also rich in minerals like calcium, magnesium, zinc, iron, selenium and potassium.

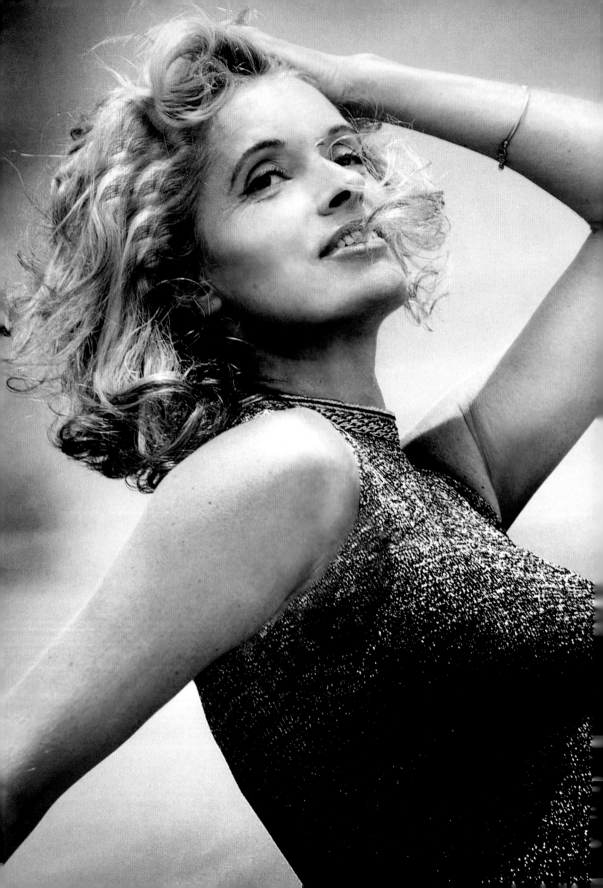

> I firmly believe that you are as young as your self-belief, as wise as your words, as old as your doubts and as beautiful as the love you hold in your heart - GREGORY LANDSMAN

I have enjoyed working with Isabella for the past seven years. Her face is synonymous with the decadence and glamour of the 1980s and she is the model Elle McPherson said she most wanted to be like. Isabella is one of the most celebrated faces in fashion and one of the few models to have graced the cover of *Vogue* six times. At fifty-three her energy and outlook on life is exemplary. At 11am sharp there is a knock on the door, she is working with me.

Isabella is an incredible role model to the beauty industry and women in general, reminding them that they can age naturally.

Face to face with *I* supermodel Isabella Cowan

Her beauty is still recognisable more than 30 years after her first *Vogue* cover went to print, but that is largely because she is comfortable in her skin.

For someone who made a career in a youth obsessed industry she conveys the relaxed air of one who is untroubled by her age. We chat about a variety of life's gifts, from love to friendship to her favourite food – spaghetti!

Her philosophy on life comes shining through her Italian accent and makes everything sound charming, even the word 'marinara'.

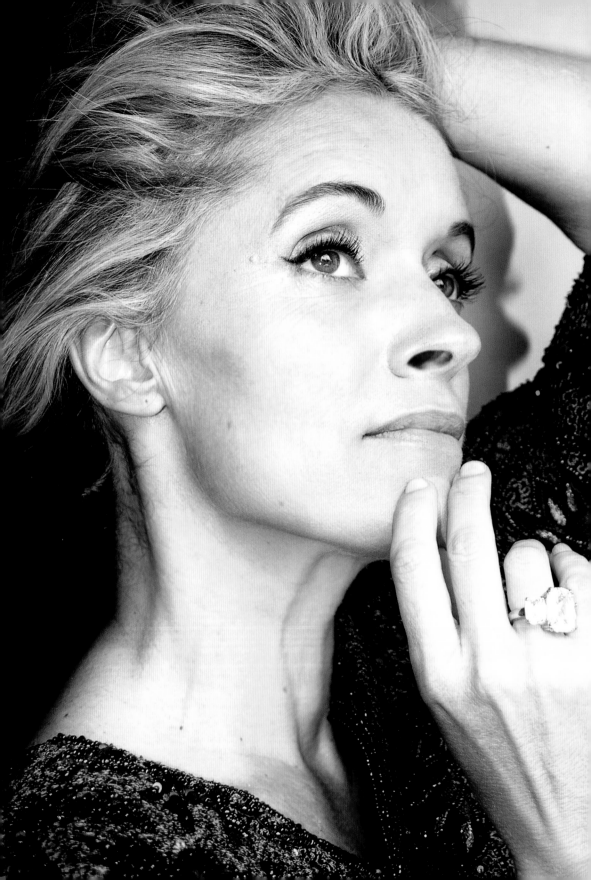

"I have always believed in a wholesome and natural approach as I learnt while I was modelling that what I ate in combination with what I put on my face made the difference to my skin in front of the camera. And so to this day I eat good quality, home cooked food to give my skin and body the vitamins and minerals it needs, and use natural skincare on my face. I don't like to eat a lot of junk food, and so I don't believe in putting the equivalent on my face!"

She operates on what I firmly believe in: the 80/20 rule.

As she declares, "I love great coffee and a glass of cold sauvignon blanc. In fact I am a great fan of practising 'Dolce far niente', the sweetness of doing nothing."

When I ask her about regrets in life she tells me that she doesn't really have any. One of her favourite

"I have so many beautiful female friends who are always criticising themselves for not being thin enough, young enough, pretty enough or sexy enough. We need to relax and let ourselves just be."

What always stands out is that Isabella is the first to laugh at herself and despite all the accolades and success she never takes herself too seriously. She laughs to herself and her laughter is spirited and infectious. In that moment I am reminded that wherever there is joy, beauty is close by.

"As women we need to do what we can do to live a happy and healthy life and then forget about it and enjoy whatever life has to offer at the time!

"To me this means living life day to day and enjoying the small things that life has to offer. After all life is made up of small things that we can choose

BEAUTY IS NOT AN AGE BUT A JOURNEY TO CELEBRATE WHO YOU ARE TODAY, LET YOUR PAST GUIDE YOU, AND THE ESSENCE OF YOUR BEAUTY INSPIRE YOU. — GREGORY LANDSMAN

quotes is that it is better to look back on life and say, 'I can't believe I did that', than to look back and say 'I wish I had!'

Of course life has had its challenges. She has survived a break up with the father of her children after 22 years, and more recently the death of her 18 year old Labrador Murphy, who travelled all over the world with her. "At these times it is easy to let life bury you, but I once read something that we should all learn from our dogs… No matter what 'crappy' situations life brings you, kick some grass over it and move on!"

She shares in my belief that many women feel significant pressure around how to manage the ageing process and that they are too hard on themselves.

to enjoy or miss while worrying constantly about something! I have done this at times, but I know every day when I get up that I have the choice to miss the best parts of my life by 'stressing', or to live fully by enjoying what I have in that moment."

I am reminded of the Dalai Lama quote:

There are only two days in the year that you cannot do anything about. One is called yesterday and the other is called tomorrow, so today is the right day to love, believe, do and mostly live.

Looking at Bella through the lens of the camera you can see that a life well lived shows up on your face. Her beauty goes well beyond her bone structure, and has so much more to do with the structure of her thoughts and the way she lives her life.

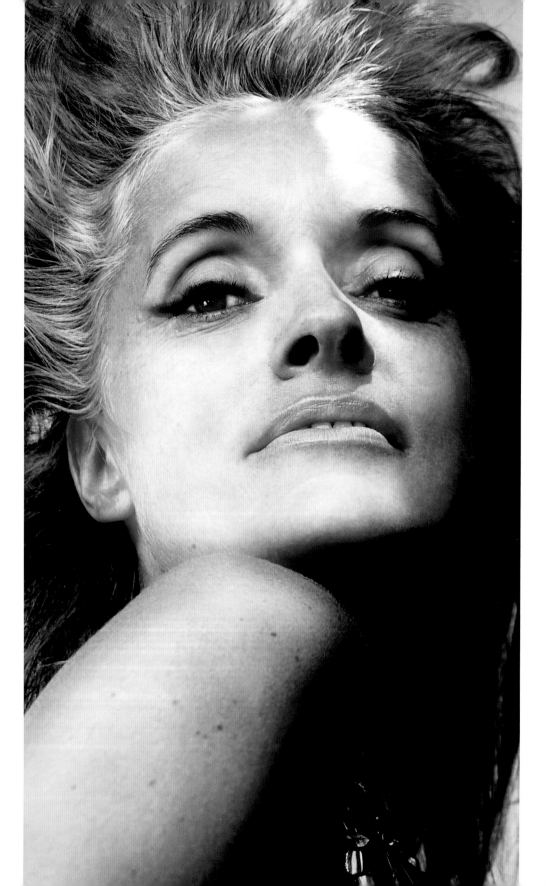

As the sun rises, let me start the day with an intention
to feel beautiful and happy.

I know that there will always be times when we feel
challenged by the world's concept of beauty.

Times when we feel that deeply cherished thoughts
about what we thought made us

valuable and

beautiful

must be left behind.

Give me the strength and courage to do this,
so that I can choose to believe in the truth
of who I am and find it in myself again.

Allow me to understand that this is the time
to create a new vision of myself.

Let this vision be born from the wisdom
of knowing my beauty as a human being.

- GREGORY LANDSMAN

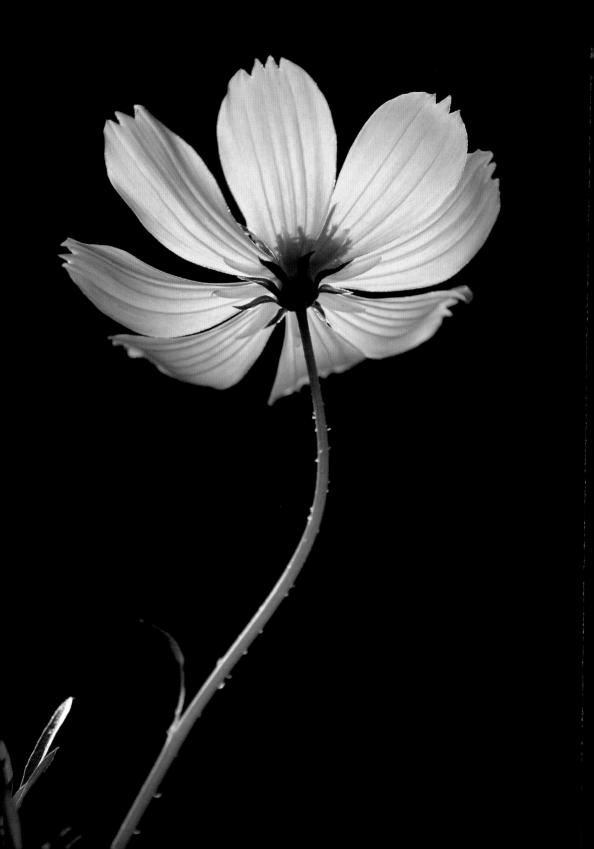

DE-STRESS WITH SKIN BUILDING VITAMINS & MINERALS

Give your skin a break from the stress of everyday life with natural face lifting vitamin and mineral formulas

While it is impossible to escape the toxins that come from everyday living we can give our skin a break with natural face lifting vitamin and mineral formulas.

Decades of experience has taught me that when it comes to getting the skin results you are looking for you can't beat powerful ingredients from nature.

A daily dose of pure vitamins and minerals delivered in a way that the skin can absorb can take years off your face.

STHEkin

The skin is the body's largest organ and two of its core functions are:

1. To create a barrier for the body – keeping moisture in and germs and toxins out; and
2. Detoxification – ridding the body of toxins.

We continue to absorb toxins through daily life (cosmetics, weather, pollution etc) and without an active plan to 'detox' and freshen our skin, the long-term impact is often dull looking skin and premature ageing.

I firmly believe that to support our skin to be as healthy as it can be we need to look at the inside and the outside to get the benefit of topical skin treatments, while looking closely at what we eat.

A glowing, healthy complexion stems from healthy skin cells, and my combined approach of treatments and good food choices to 'de-stress' can help your skin become stronger and more resilient, retain moisture and ultimately look younger and stay younger. There is no need to worry, it isn't complicated and regardless of your age it isn't too late to start.

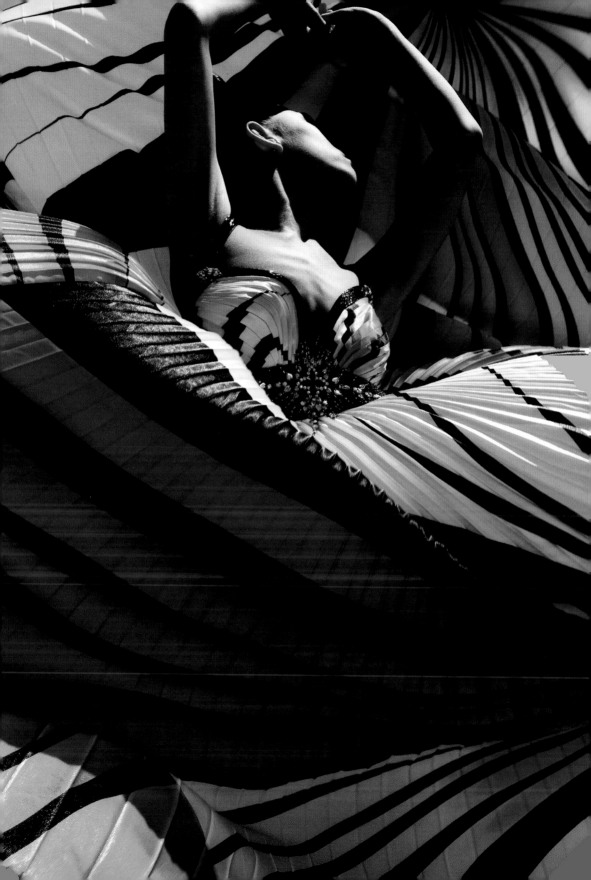

GET skin fit!

It's all in the science! Tips on where to find essential skin builders

Having being privileged to work alongside chemists creating skin care, I know that you can achieve amazing results with the purity of nature.

Alpha hydroxy acid (AHA) acts as a natural exfoliant that removes dead skin cells and leaves skin healthier and renewed. AHA can be found in a number of foods and plants in different forms including glycolic acid, malic acid, lactic acid and citric acid.

Glycolic acid is one of the most effective AHAs used for skin exfoliation, oil reduction, collagen building and skin bleaching. It can be found in sugar (from sugar cane) and unripened grapes.

Lactic acid gently exfoliates and softens the skin and can be found in dairy products.

Malic acid is also good for skin exfoliation and can be found in nectarines, bananas, cherries, blackberries, apples, pears and grapes.

Citric acid is an antioxidant used for collagen building and skin bleaching. Citric acid is also a beta hydroxy acid, which means it has the ability to cut through grease and oil on the skin. Citric acid can be found in lemons, limes, oranges, pineapples, grapefruits and berries.

Vitamin A (made up of retinol and carotene) renews skin through the stimulation of elastin and collagen production, resulting in smoother, more elastic skin. It has also been shown to remove fine lines, help repair sun damaged skin and reduce age spots. Vitamin A is found in egg yolk, milk and other dairy products, fish, fish oil, sweet potato, carrot, raw spinach, raw tomato, papaya, apricot, broccoli, orange and cantaloupe.

When it comes to skin care there is a lot of confusion, but if you want clear, radiant skin, you can't go past *Mother Nature's* nutrients

Vitamin B3	helps regulate oil secretion and decreases a pre-disposition to blemishes. It can prevent dermatitis and scaly skin and is known as an acne treatment. It can be found in cranberries, tomatoes and green peas.
Vitamin B5	helps to increase moisture content in hair and skin. Vitamin B5 is found in cranberries, sunflower seeds and tomatoes.
Vitamin C	is known to stimulate collagen production, which gives the skin elasticity. It helps neutralise free radical activity, protects against UVA/UVB rays and helps heal scar tissue and bruising.
Vitamin C	can be found in citrus fruits, peaches, strawberries, cranberries, mangoes, green and red peppers, papaya, pineapple, grapes, mustard greens, broccoli, cabbage, spinach, tomatoes, fortified cereals, berries, melons, potatoes, kiwi, guava, peas, sweet potato and parsley.
Vitamin D	has strong moisturising properties and encourages tissue development. Vitamin D can be found in egg yolk, salmon, liver, herring, fortified milk and sunflower oil.
Vitamin E	is known to condition and moisturise the skin, inhibit free radical damage and help heal scars. Vitamin E can be found in wheat germ, nuts, sunflower seeds, vegetable oil (including olive, safflower, sunflower), green leafy vegetables, tomatoes and whole grains.

ANTIOXIDANT
skin·firming
TREATMENT

Banana and oatmeal skin firming treatment

You will need:

- ½ banana with the skin on
- 2 tablespoons wheat flour
- 2 tablespoons oatmeal
- 1 tablespoon blackstrap molasses
- 1 tablespoon mineral water

How to make it:

1. Cut the banana with the skin on into small slices and add to a blender along with all the other ingredients. Mix it just enough so you get a nice sticky paste that you can apply to your face without it running off.

2. Add more oatmeal if needed to get the right consistency.

3. Spread the paste gently and equally with your fingertips on your clean face and neck, making sure to keep the eye area clear.

4. Lie down, relax and leave the mask on for 5-10 minutes.

5. Wash the mask off with warm water and end with a splash of cold water. Finally, apply moisturiser to your damp face.

THE GL SKINFIT SECRET THAT DELIVERS REAL RESULTS

Banana peels contain high amounts of certain vitamins that are important to human health, including vitamins A and B6. Vitamin A helps renew skin through the stimulation of elastin and collagen production resulting in smoother more elastic skin. Blackstrap molasses is rich in minerals and vitamins like iron, calcium, potassium, magnesium, copper and vitamin B6, essential for skin development. The high copper content stimulates the production of elastin to strengthen, firm and smooth skin. Copper also serves as an antioxidant to protect skin from stress and improve the barrier function of the skin.

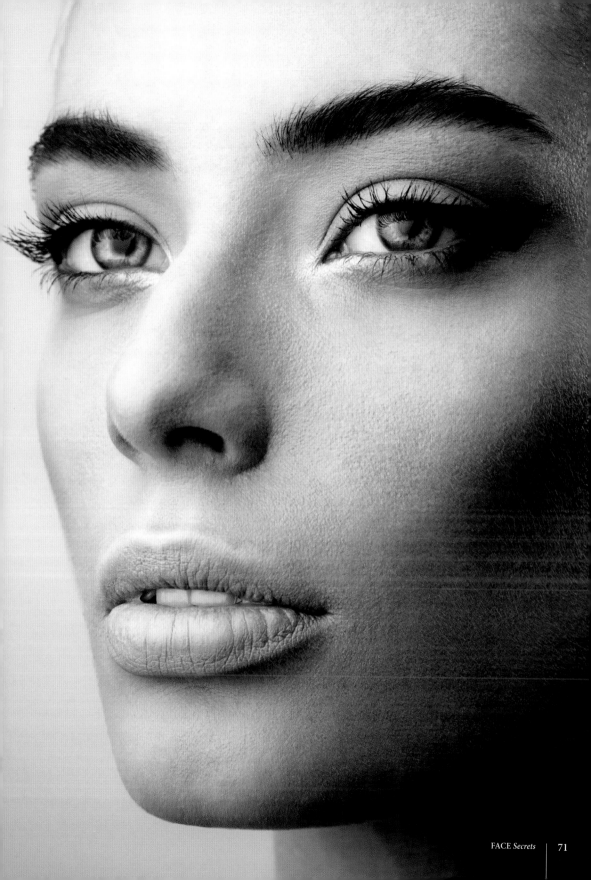

UNDER EYE skin. brightening TREATMENT

Potato skin brightening treatment

You will need:

- 1 potato

How to make it:

1. Run the potato through a food processor or juicer and place the raw potato pulp into a piece of clean cloth, squeeze the juice into a container. If using a juicer, dip cotton balls straight into the potato juice and discard the pulp.

2. Using cotton balls, apply the juice from the potato directly beneath your eyes, but do not let it come into contact with the eye itself.

3. For best results leave on for 30 minutes then wash your face with warm water. Apply regularly.

THE GL SKINFIT SECRET THAT DELIVERS REAL RESULTS

The secret in potatoes is an enzyme called catecholase, which is used in many cosmetics as a skin brightener.

Beauty truths

We all have our own
definition of beauty but
when it comes to the truth
of beauty, for me it is
looking into the depth of our
heart and celebrating who
we are inside, expressing
ourselves fully and letting
our uniqueness shine.

- GREGORY LANDSMAN

ALL CLEAR

END FREAK OUTS AND

break outs

Secrets to skin renewal for problem spots

Our skin does a lot to support us; it protects us, warms us and transmits the loving touch of our loved ones. So it makes sense to show it some tender loving care when it breaks out. This face treatment feels like a spa treatment but works its magic on blemishes.

Banana face nourisher to counteract blemishes

You will need:

- 2 egg yolks
- 1 cup (250ml) olive oil
- 1 banana

How to make it:

1. Beat the egg yolks and olive oil until thoroughly mixed.

2. Mash a ripe banana and add it to the mixture.

3. Apply the mixture over the face and neck and leave for 30 minutes.

4. Rinse the mixture off with cold water.

THE GL SKINFIT SECRET THAT DELIVERS REAL RESULTS

This treatment nourishes your skin with a cocktail of antioxidants, vitamins A (retinol), D, B5, E and K, antibacterial properties and sulphur to counteract blemishes and assist in restoring collagen.

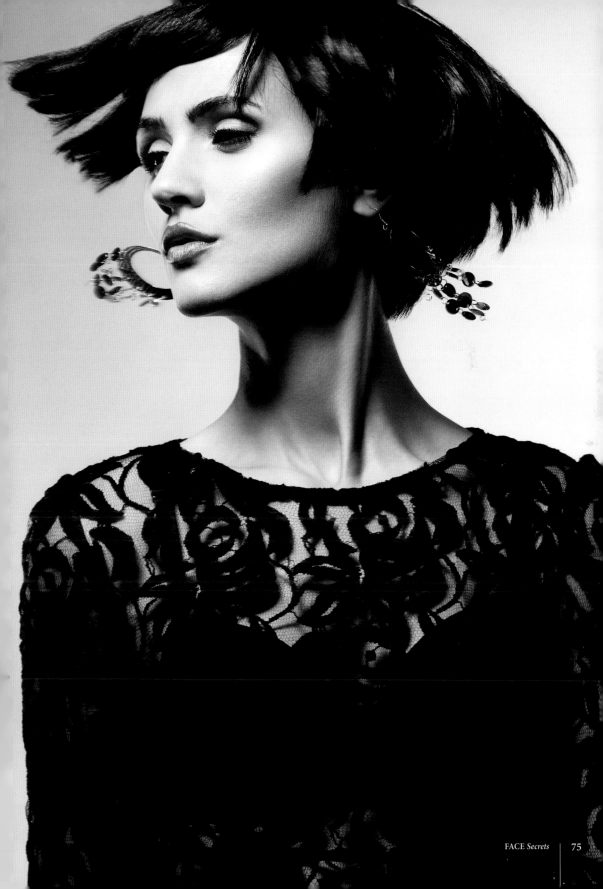

THE PRAYER OF
choice

It has taken many years to understand

That if I believe I am ugly I will know ugliness

If I believe my body is not perfect I will know imperfection

If I believe I am beautiful

I will know beauty

This is my power to choose what I believe

Guide my thoughts so I can choose carefully

- GREGORY LANDSMAN

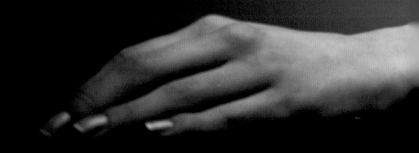

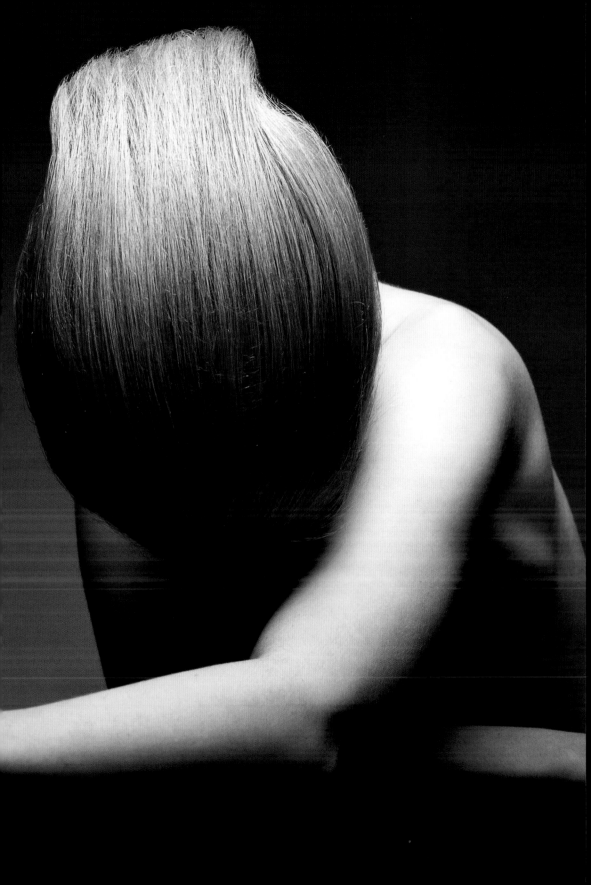

ANTIOXIDANT EXFOLIATING body scrub

TO DETOX AND DE-STRESS

If you want to get the most out of your moisturiser and enjoy soft, smooth and glowing skin then this treatment is for you. Toxic accumulation and poor circulation can create a loss of firmness in the skin. This treatment stimulates, exfoliates and speeds up the lymphatic drainage system to remove toxins. So if you haven't been exercising enough and feel you need a boost then this treatment is for you.

Ginger and cinnamon body scrub

You will need:

- 1 medium sized ginger nugget
- ½ tablespoon cinnamon
- 1 cup sea salt
- 1 lemon, juiced
- Organic grape seed oil

How to make it:

1. Grate the ginger nugget then squeeze the juice from it into a bowl.

2. Add ½ tablespoon of the freshly grated ginger root.

3. Add the cinnamon, sea salt, lemon juice and grape seed oil and mix together.

4. Gently rub the mixture in circular motions all over your body and face. This will speed up the lymphatic drainage system while exfoliating the skin, leaving it hydrated, supple and soft.

THE GL SKINFIT SECRET THAT DELIVERS REAL RESULTS

Cinnamon has five times as many antioxidants as ½ cup of blueberries, so it is a great free radical fighter. Ginger contains the powerful antioxidant gingerol that protects and stimulates skin, which makes it ideal for skin treatments. Lemons give skin a good dose of alpha hydroxy acid, which stimulates collagen and elastin and helps remove dead skin cells to reveal fresh new skin. The vitamin E in the grape seed oil helps repair skin.

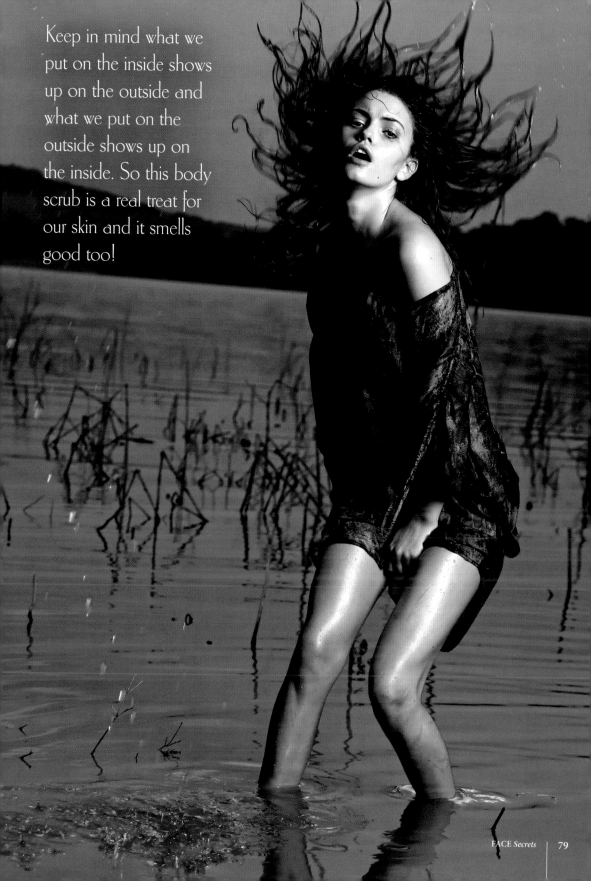

Keep in mind what we put on the inside shows up on the outside and what we put on the outside shows up on the inside. So this body scrub is a real treat for our skin and it smells good too!

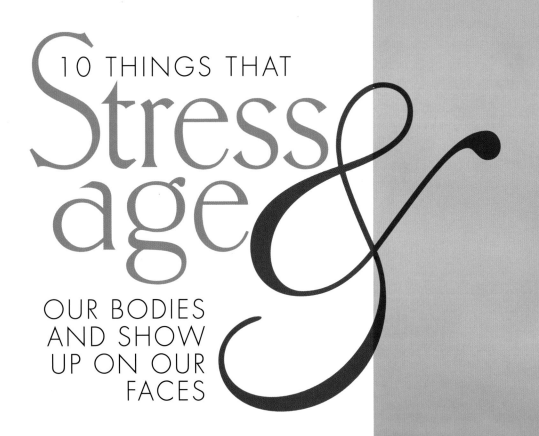

10 THINGS THAT
Stress & age
OUR BODIES AND SHOW UP ON OUR FACES

While genetic factors play a major role in the way we age, so does our lifestyle.

In our health conscious society, the words "You look stressed" are all too familiar. If we are not saying them to ourselves, we are saying them to others.

Here are 10 things (in no particular order) that contribute to ageing and stress being stored in our bodies and showing up on our faces.

1. Excess alcohol
2. Mental anxiety
3. Smoking and drugs
4. Low exercise
5. Saturated fats
6. Unprotected or excessive sun exposure
7. Polluted air
8. Not enough sleep
9. Excess weight
10. Sugar consumption

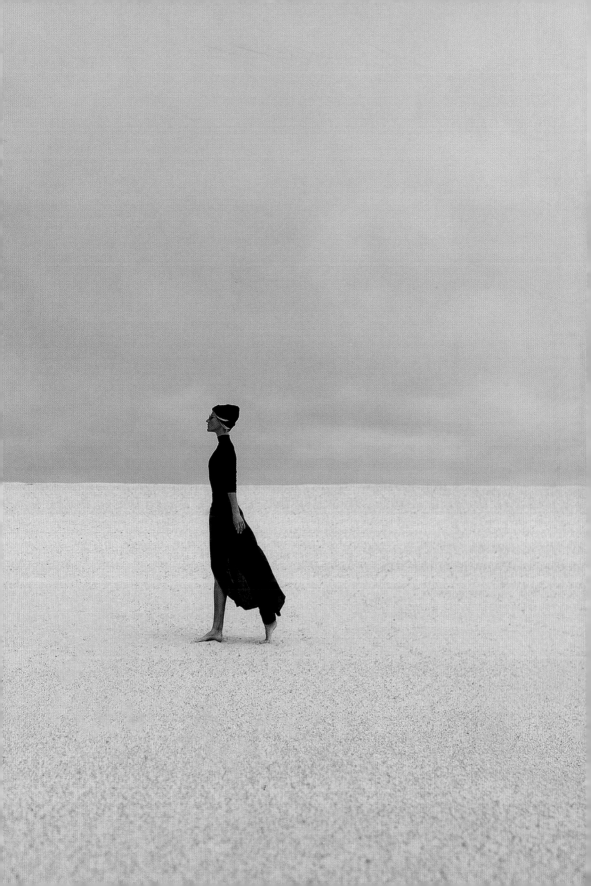

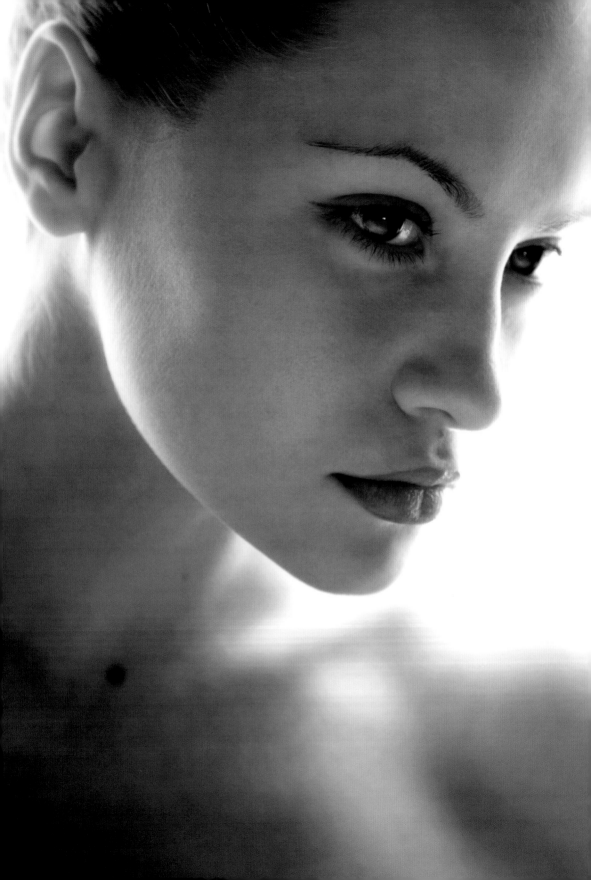

FUEL YOUR SKIN WITH

face lifting food

Food is a powerful transformational element that we can use to help de-stress the skin and achieve tighter and more youthful looking skin.

Beauty Truth

There is something about fresh and simplistic food that gives you honest flavours and nutrients and this collagen boosting chicken recipe is full of both!

Keep in mind that all of the high price skin-care products that include retinol and retinoic acid are actually derived from vitamin A, which supports our skin's elastin, and sweet potatoes are full of it. They also contain beta-carotene and vitamin C. To get the most out of them from a health point of view, don't peel them as there is a lot of goodness in the skin.

In addition, these little beauties contain vitamin E, which helps the body regenerate vitamin C, along with potassium to help us relax during stressful times.

There's a lot of nutritional power in this potato! In fact one might even go as far as to say that they are a super skin food!

Your skin is like life; you only get out of it what you put in.

Collagen boosting chicken with sweet potato and horseradish salad

You will need:

- 1kg/2.2 lb sweet potatoes, cut into little chunks
- 1 red/Spanish onion
- 6 tablespoons olive oil
- 4 tablespoons coriander/cilantro
- ¾ cup plus 1 tablespoon (200ml) unsweetened yoghurt
- 4 tablespoons horseradish

- ½ teaspoon English mustard
- 1 teaspoon black peppercorns
- 6 chicken drumsticks
- 4 garlic cloves
- ½ cup (125ml) white wine
- Handful of parsley

How to make it:

1. Sweet potatoes bring a lot of sweetness to our skin. Boil the potatoes in water until they are just tender, but don't overdo it as you don't want them soft and mushy. Drain the potatoes and place them in a bowl.

2. Peel and slice the onion and add to a pan with 3 tablespoons of olive oil over low heat, sauté until soft and golden.

3. Gently crush the coriander leaves and add to the onion. This herb makes everything come alive whether you use it in a curry, a salad or a soup. When the onion is done remove it from the pan and set aside.

4. In a separate bowl, mix the yoghurt with the horseradish and mustard. Pour over the potato and gently mix it through.

5. Crush the black peppercorns and quick fry in a dry pan for two minutes to unleash all the flavour.

6. Pour three tablespoons of oil into the pan and add the chicken drumsticks. Brown the drumsticks, turning them as they gain colour. Cook for 15 minutes.

7. Crush the garlic and add it to the pan along with the wine and cooked onion. Let it cook slowly over a low heat until the drumsticks are cooked through. Including garlic in the recipe adds nutrients and the sulphur in it helps our bodies produce collagen. When the drumsticks are cooked through, you are ready to plate it up.

8. Place a serve of potatoes on the bottom and top with two or three drumsticks per person. Garnish with chopped parsley.

THE GL SKINFIT SECRET THAT DELIVERS REAL RESULTS

Sweet potato is loaded with vitamin A, which supports elastin and keeps skin nice and firm. Horseradish has an exceptionally high vitamin C content, which helps boost our collagen production and fight the free radicals that cause premature ageing.

Let my beauty miraculously unfold inside of me

Let it unfold outside of me and below me

Let it dance beside me and around me

So I can experience the momentum of it

The importance of it

And the eternal

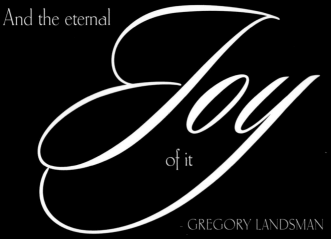

Joy

of it

— GREGORY LANDSMAN

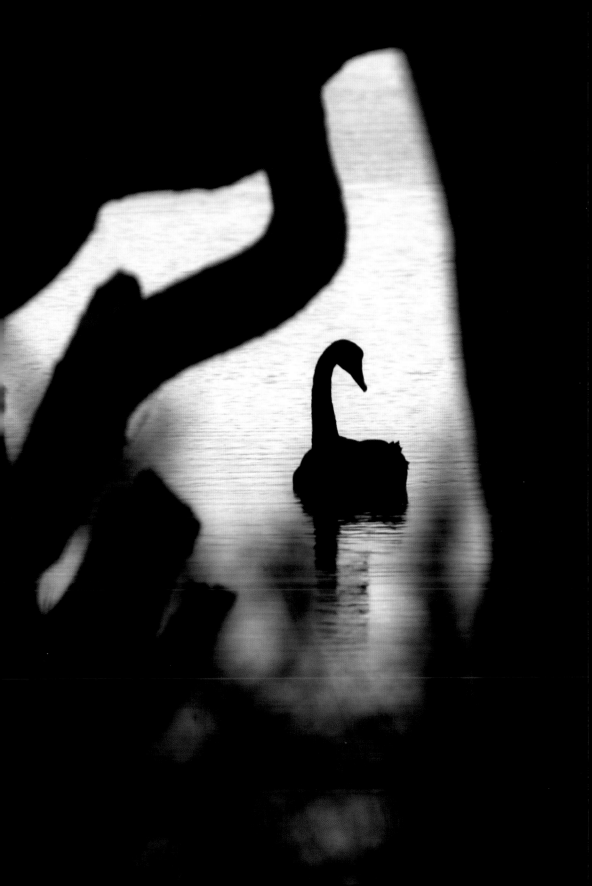

Skin boosting sesame seed
tuna with vegetables and tahini sauce

Tuna is a good source of omega-3 fatty acids, which work hard to moisturise our skin from the inside out and naturally plumps out fine lines.

You will need:

- 12 tablespoons sesame seeds
- 2 tuna steaks
- Handful of French green beans
- 1 zucchini/courgette
- 1 punnet of cherry tomatoes
- 5 tablespoons lemon juice
- 2 tablespoons tahini
- Grape seed oil
- 1 tablespoon water

How to make it:

1. Fry the sesame seeds in a dry pan then coat the raw tuna steaks in the seeds and put aside.

2. To prepare the salad, cut up the green beans and slice the zucchini. Place them in a steamer along with the cherry tomatoes. The tomatoes are sweet and delicious, but also rich in the antioxidant lycopene, which inhibits collagenases – enzymes that destroy collagen. However, the lycopene is only accessed when tomatoes are cooked. Tomatoes are loaded with vitamins C, A and E, which stimulates our collagen and elastin and keeps skin smooth.

3. To make the dressing, mix the lemon juice and tahini. Add the grape seed oil and water and mix into a nice paste. Place to the side while you cook the tuna steaks.

4. Heat a pan with some grape seed oil over a medium heat. Once the pan is heated place the steaks in it. Try not to turn the steaks more than once so that you don't overcook them. Cook for approximately 3 minutes on each side for rare to medium. (Personally I like it medium rare but I know others like it well done.)

5. Toss the vegetable mix with 2 tablespoons of grapeseed oil, add lemon zest and a squeeze of lemon juice to give an extra nutrient boost.

6. Place the steaks on top of the vegetables and add a dollop of the tahini and lemon sauce.

THE GL SKINFIT SECRET THAT DELIVERS REAL RESULTS

Tuna is a good source of omega-3 fatty acids, which naturally plumps out fine lines. Tahini is a powerhouse of vitamins and is loaded with vitamins E, B1, B2, B3, B5, B6, B15, biotin and choline. It is also a source of vitamin A. This ingredient is full of everything that is good for our skin.

The *fountain* of youth lies in Mother Nature's vitamins and minerals that strengthen and *protect* our skin.

You have got to love fresh fruit and vegetables!

Antioxidant chocolate fondue dessert

If you are feeling like something sweet, and let's face it most of us do, this dessert is a winner on every level. This dessert is full of nutrients like potassium, magnesium, vitamins B1, B2, D and E, as well as serotonin, a neurotransmitter that acts as an anti-depressant. But it is also 'choc full' of flavonoids that protect our skin and keep it soft.

You will need:

- 1 large banana
- 1 cup (250ml) water
- 340g/12 oz dark chocolate
- 4 large oranges/2 cups (500ml) orange juice
- 2 teaspoons cinnamon
- 1 punnet of ripe strawberries
- A fondue heating pot

How to make it:

1. Blend the banana and water together. Place the mixture in a saucepan on low and let it heat slowly.

2. Zest the oranges and add it to the sauce.

3. Squeeze the oranges to get 2 cups (500ml) of juice. The juice gives the dessert a tangy citrus taste that brings a lot of freshness to the sauce. Add the juice to the pan and heat slowly over low.

4. Add the chocolate and melt it into the mixture gently, ensuring it doesn't burn. Add the cinnamon for an extra antioxidant boost.

5. Run the strawberries under water, dry them gently and then thread the fruit onto skewers.

6. Add the chocolate sauce to a fondue pot and place the skewers on a tray to serve. Turn on the heat to keep the sauce warm and you are ready to eat and dip!

THE GL SKINFIT SECRET THAT DELIVERS REAL RESULTS

Strawberries contain vitamins C and B and combined with the antioxidants are essential for the structure of collagen and elastin that supports the elasticity and firmness of our skin. Dark chocolate is full of nutrients such as potassium, magnesium, vitamins B1, B2, D and E and is loaded with flavonoids that protect our skin and keep it soft.

To be true to your beauty

You must be true to your

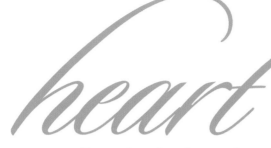

heart

From this day forward

Never excuse who you are

Reach out

Touch life with your body

Embrace life with your mind

Remember beauty with your thoughts

Feel it with your heart

Start to live it

beauty

is your birth right

Claim it

- GREGORY LANDSMAN

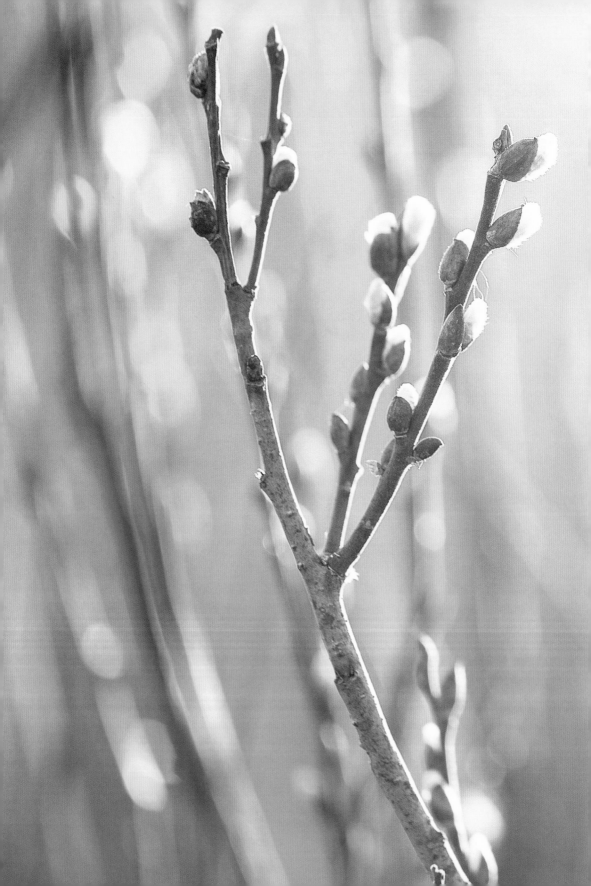

FACE SECRETS TO LIFT, TRANSFORM AND REJUVENATE

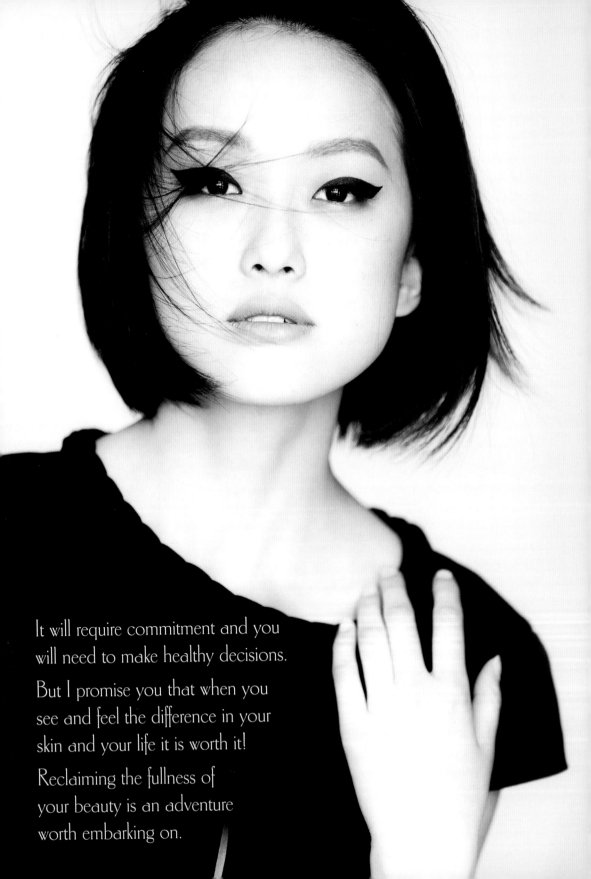

It will require commitment and you
will need to make healthy decisions.

But I promise you that when you
see and feel the difference in your
skin and your life it is worth it!

Reclaiming the fullness of
your beauty is an adventure
worth embarking on.

Train your brain and build stronger, younger looking skin... what you think you will feel, and what you feel you will create and see on your face.

In the work that I do, whenever I touch a face I experience over and over the honesty that sits on our faces as our skin never lies. It is like a compass guiding us to understand our inner world. The face reveals it all ... the stress we feel, the worry that is silently carried, the sleep that is missed, the meals that were not eaten, even the water we haven't drunk.

And when I ask women across the world how they feel about their skin and the way they look, more often than not they give me a list of what is wrong and what they don't have. I hear that their skin is dry and sagging, they have wrinkles appearing, they don't know what to do with their neck or hands and that they believe they are 'ageing before their eyes'!

And therein lies the link between our faces and what we feel. When things are going wrong in our lives or we feel critical and unhappy about something, it creates lots of small almost unnoticeable stresses that build up until one day we realise that our stresses and the way we think are sitting on our faces.

RECLAIMING
beauty

It is easy to focus on what is wrong with us, to see the faults as opposed to the beauty. But gravitating towards what needs fixing blinds us to what is truly good and beautiful.

Most people never see themselves as beautiful. But having worked with women of all ages, I can say with certainty that I have never met a woman who does not possess beauty. Regardless of who you are, how old you are or where you come from, you can feel beautiful!

Focusing on our goodness becomes an unstoppable force that ensures we know our value. But more often than not it requires us to open our eyes as well as our hearts. If we only use our eyes to see our beauty we will only ever see the smallest aspects of what makes us truly beautiful. The most beautiful gifts we posses are only ever revealed to us when we are willing to have the courage to look beyond our physical bodies and our material lives to what lies beneath.

If at this point you are saying to yourself: I am too old; it will never work for me; it might have worked if I was younger, then these are the excuses that can stop you from experiencing and seeing the beauty of who you are.

The books I write and the products I develop are all born out of years of working with models (and include what I practice myself) and all work to do the same thing: de-stress your skin and your life so you can look younger, feel younger and stay younger.

But before we get started you need to acknowledge that ... YOU CAN DO IT.

face lifting

EXERCISES

It's not wrinkles that change the shape of the face with age, but sagging muscles & skin!

Why a natural lift works!

Every major muscle on the face can be shaped and strengthened. And like any other muscle in the body, if muscles are not exercised, they will become weak and begin to sag. These techniques strengthen the muscles, supporting the skin to be tight and toned while reducing and softening wrinkles – a truly healthy preventative against skin ageing.

Why face lifting exercises last longer than any face lift

Unlike the rest of the body, where muscles are attached to bones, facial muscles are attached directly to the skin. This means that as the muscles weaken, skin sags and the face drops.

Face-lifts are designed to tighten the skin by disconnecting the muscles from the skin and then pulling and stitching them higher on the face. The trouble is that because a muscle isn't exercised, even after it has been surgically pulled, it will eventually sag once again. It simply has to, as the only long term solution we have to fight gravity on our faces or our bodies is exercise!

Yet while we are busy eliminating the stress from the muscles in our body, we often neglect the fifty-seven muscles in our face.

We seem to take it for granted that we can smile, sneeze, laugh, yawn and express our feelings with our faces, but we pay little or no attention to the facial muscles that make this possible.

OUR GENES / ARE NOT.
our destiny
AND THE WAY OUR FACES AGE /
IS LITERALLY IN OUR HANDS

I wrote the book *Face Fitness* to show that exercising and conditioning the face will outlast and outperform any surgical face-lift or artificial face fillers enabling us to address the following:

- Drain toxins that age the skin
- Prevent and reduce wrinkles without anaesthetic
- Sculpt and reshape the face without pain
- Minimise lines around the mouth without collagen
- Lift sagging skin without stitches
- Reduce crow's feet and the folds in the upper and lower eyelids without a surgeon
- Minimise a double chin without cutting
- Tighten jowls and loose skin on the neck without the expense
- Plump up hollow cheeks without face fillers, and
- Oxygenate the blood to give your skin a lasting healthy glow.

So regardless of your age, your level of stress or whether you have had a face lift or not, exercising just 10 minutes a day can help you regain and retain strong facial muscles that will support the skin to stay firm and healthy. It only takes 10 minutes a day.

Releasing stress from the facial muscles

Massage speeds up lymphatic drainage, which removes toxins and de-stresses the muscles on the face and neck that cause crow's feet, wrinkled lips, a sagging jaw line, and heavy jowls and frown lines.

Things you need to know...

- Before you start, rub your hands together vigorously and place over the face to energise.
- Oil is required to provide a thin surface for hands to glide over, so the skin is not pulled or stretched.
- When doing the exercises, work upwards. This way the veins benefit most from the blood circulation created through this process.
- Start with a slow speed and increase the speed as you go, ensuring that the skin has only slight pressure placed on it.
- Be aware that as you do the exercises your skin may appear red or slightly blotchy immediately afterwards. This simply shows that it is working and that there is additional circulation in the area.
- As you go through the routine, breathe deeply and slowly and you will feel your facial muscles relax. Let each breath empower you and let go of the stress and tension.

7 secrets TO *banish*

FOREHEAD WORRY LINES

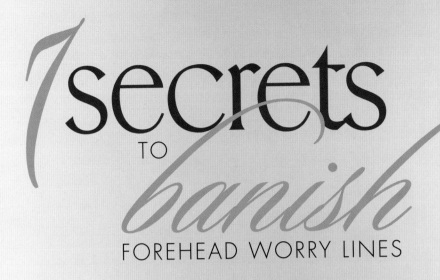

Combining Face Fitness massage with skin treatments is a dynamic way to deal with forehead worry lines.

There is no doubt about it that lifestyle, habits, dooming headlines and environmental stresses all take a toll on our skin. But here are numerous natural treatments to hydrate, counteract, remove and prevent worry lines and home remedies to obtain a smoother, firmer, younger forehead.

1. Rub a slice of lemon over your forehead every morning and every night or alternate with cucumber.
2. Apply moisturiser or night serum and give your face and forehead a good massage. This speeds up the lymphatic drainage system and oxygenates the blood.
3. Take 1 tablespoon of fresh flaxseed oil or fish oil capsules 4 times a day, as they moisturise the skin from the inside out.
4. For a quick skin boost rub an ice cube over your forehead furrows. This improves blood circulation and prevents forehead lines.
5. Ensure you use sun protection and avoid smoking.
6. Drinking a minimum of 8-10 glasses of water a day helps hydrates the skin and flush toxins from our system that age the skin.
7. Use three fingers to rub the forehead upwards from the brows to the hairline in a continuous movement.

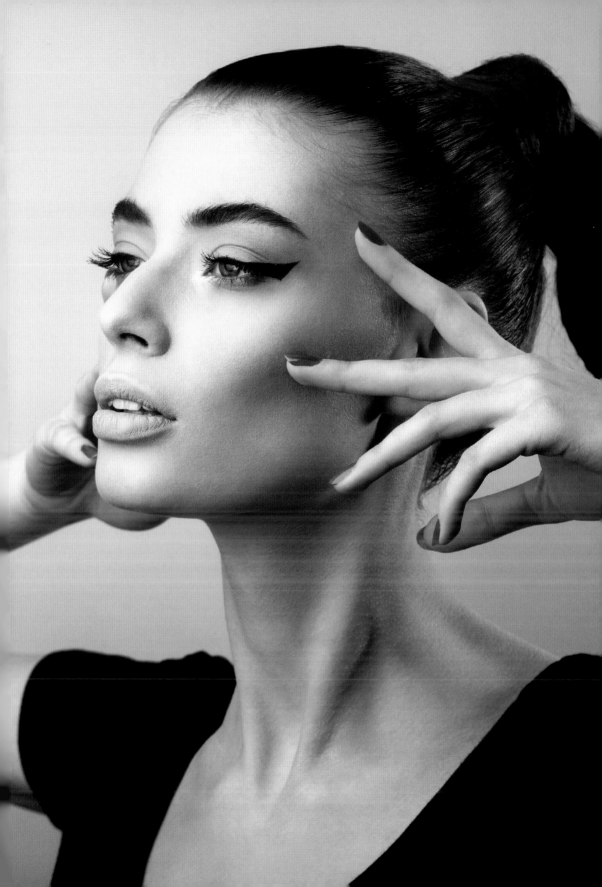

wrinkle

FREE

lips

PREVENTING LINES AROUND THE MOUTH

Tighten lip muscles

Lip exercises tone the muscles in your face, which may reduce lip wrinkles and signs of facial sagging. Eliminate wrinkles around mouth and keep your lips looking plump using these face exercises for your mouth.

Lip lock

This action strengthens and tightens the muscle around the mouth, smoothing out lines and enlarging lips for a fuller, firmer look.

1. Place the index finger from each hand inside the corners of the mouth and pull the mouth wide at the corners.
2. Pull the fingers back together then release and pull wide once again. Repeat 15 times.

TIP To get your lips SKINFIT don't pull too hard on the mouth when it is wide, as this will stress the muscle. The stretch to be achieved here is gentle and the contraction of the mouth pulls the fingers together. Don't forget to maintain steady breathing.

THE GL SKINFIT SECRET THAT DELIVERS REAL RESULTS

Contracting the muscle builds fibres while simultaneously plumping the tissue. This reduces and prevents the appearance of fine lines around the mouth.

TIP Exfoliate lips once a week using a toothbrush and some olive oil to gently bring moisture to the lips and remove dead skin cells.

NECK TO NECK
toning
TREATMENT

The skin on the neck has less sebaceous glands and is much thinner so it needs some extra care to moisturise, tighten and lift it.

Neck firming

1. To tighten the neck and jaw line, apply a light coating of castor oil to the neck.
2. Place both hands side by side in front of the throat.
3. Using your fingers, push the skin on your neck firmly upward to the chin, then outward toward the ears and finally circling down toward your collarbone.
4. Repeat this movement three to four times.

Doing this simple exercise daily should result in a leaner, more toned neck within 4-6 weeks and replace the need to use expensive neck firming creams.

THE GL SKINFIT SECRET THAT DELIVERS REAL RESULTS

The secret to this treatment is in the motion, which increases skin-firming blood circulation and drains any fluid build up. The castor oil delivers triglycerides to the skin including ricinoleic acid, oleic and linoleic acids, all of which are effective in the prevention of fine lines.

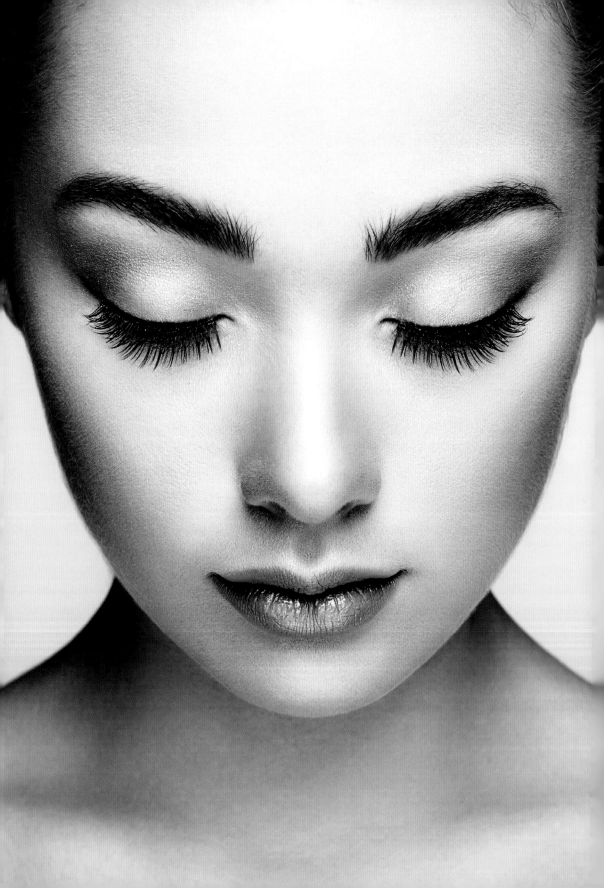

Let me use each day to exercise joyously
and do what feels good in my body

Give me the strength to run,
walk, breathe and dance

Let me make the time to pray daily

To sing loudly

To contemplate regularly

For it exercises my heart

Expresses my spirit

And allows me to remember

That there is nothing ugly
about the human body

Only the 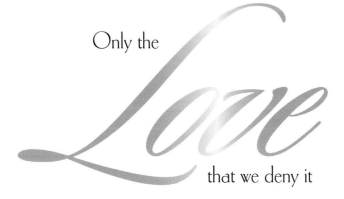 that we deny it

- GREGORY LANDSMAN

Sleep

TO FRESH 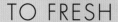 GLOWING SKIN

Not getting enough sleep is easy
to do, especially with our hectic
lifestyles, and the place that it
often shows is on our face.

When you get less than eight hours sleep it
is like trying to plan a long trip with a car
that does not have enough fuel.

A good night's sleep is one of the most
underrated beauty tools that we have at our
disposal, which is why it is something that
I put on every everyone's beauty to do list.

Sleep, sleep, sleep!

Turns out, there is a lot of meaning
behind the term 'sleeping beauty'!

THE GL SKINFIT SECRET THAT DELIVERS REAL RESULTS

Something powerful happens when we fall asleep ... we release
a youth activating hormone called the human growth hormone.
This hormone builds us up and helps create thicker skin, giving
us a more youthful appearance over all, stronger bones and
increased muscle mass. It is a part of normal tissue repair,
helping to regenerate what had been broken down
by day-to-day activities.

Sleeping beauty reminders

1. Try to get to bed by 10 p.m.
2. Stop caffeine intake at 3 p.m.
3. Have dinner at least 3 hours before you go to bed. Going to bed on a full stomach means your body spends energy digesting food as opposed to conserving it for the next day.
4. Avoid watching television before bed as it stimulates the brain.
5. Try not to consume too many fluids before you retire, so you don't have to get up in the middle of the night.
6. Turn off all electrical devices, especially your mobile telephone.
7. Apply some lavender essential oil on your pillowcase.
8. As you shut your eyes, give thanks for all the good in your life, sleep tight and keep your skin bright!

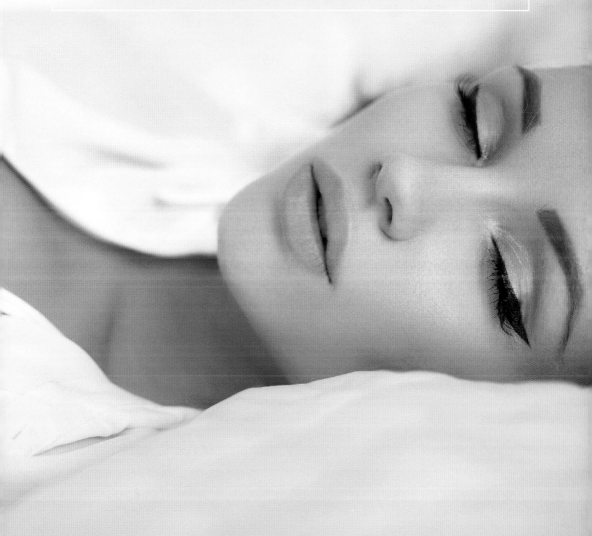

DISCOVER THE POWER

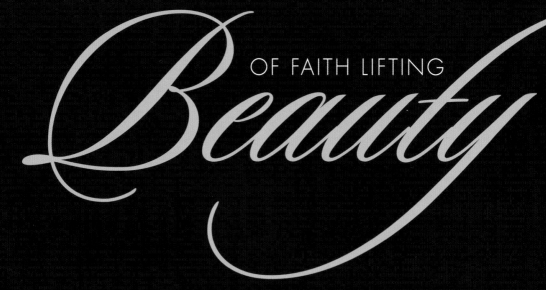

OF FAITH LIFTING

Beauty

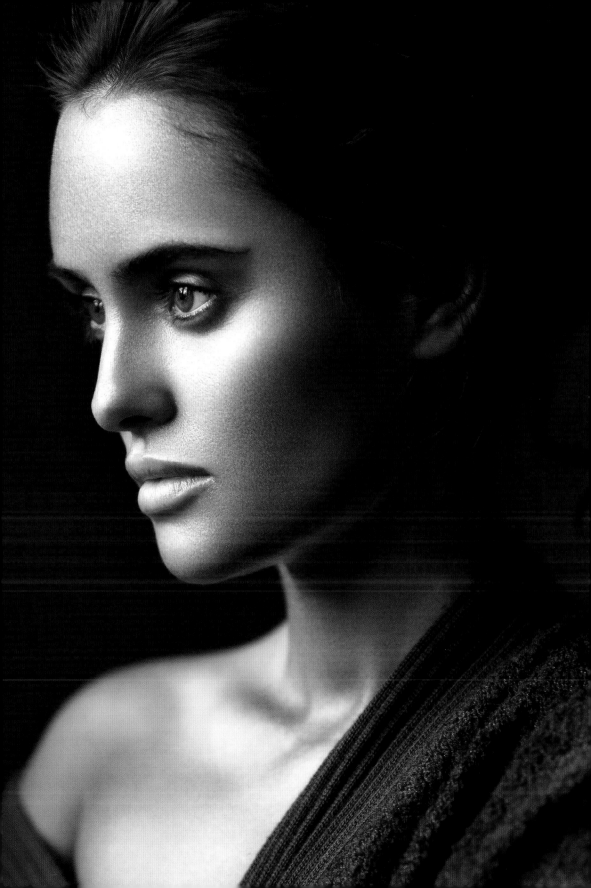

If my fifty two years on this earth have taught me anything, it is that one of the greatest challenges we face is to know our value as a human being.

Yet as human beings we are beautiful in so many extraordinary ways and just looking at how the human body functions, there is no doubt we are remarkable. So while I believe that with commitment we can do and be anything, I also believe that we are all innately beautiful.

And when we acknowledge this we break free from unrealistic expectations and false beliefs that break down our beauty feature by feature, until all we see is imperfection.

When our view of perfect beauty is an air brushed, manipulated, photoshopped image on the front of a magazine (that often bears little resemblance to the original photo) we will inevitably fall short. After all how can we compare what is not real with what is real and whole? This is a game that none of us can win at and as a result we can never experience the best version of ourselves.

Yet when we see ourselves in a full spectrum, taking in all that we are, we can see a beautiful light, recognising that our physical body is only one aspect of what makes us truly beautiful.

Accepting our beauty without isolating it to certain physical characteristics gives us the strength to no longer make our individual body parts wrong; and in doing this we acknowledge our humanity.

Every face is perfectly beautiful and unique and I often remind people that there is nothing ugly about our faces, only the love that we deny them.

Through my years in the fashion and beauty industry and my own personal experiences growing up in South Africa, I have spent countless hours asking myself: what defines beauty? My personal journey

to understand beauty resulted in a philosophy that uses the word BEAUTY as an acronym, based on the principles of: **B**alance, **E**nthusiasm, **A**cceptance, **U**nderstanding, **T**rust and **Y**ou.

This philosophy of beauty reminds me to observe the way I live, the way I love and reaffirms that laughter, fun, tears and kindness are a large part of what makes us beautiful … and our lives magical.

The principals that make up a life of BEAUTY are:

Balance

Balance is not about indulgence or repression, but in seeking balance we are encouraged to look closely at the relationship we have with ourselves so that we can begin to live in a balanced way, physically, emotionally, mentally and spiritually.

Feeling a sense of balance enables us to know that you are a divine, beautiful human being and the beauty that surrounds you, from the magnificent sunsets to a butterfly, comes from the same source that created you.

- Use your body to live your beauty, your heart to feel it, your eyes to see it, your ears to hear it, your mouth to speak it and your hands to share it.
- Practice wholeness - eat and exercise to increase the flow of energy and nurture wholesome emotions.
- Breathe deeply, it supports your nervous system to relax and helps alleviate anxiety.
- Never settle for less than you know in your heart you really deserve.

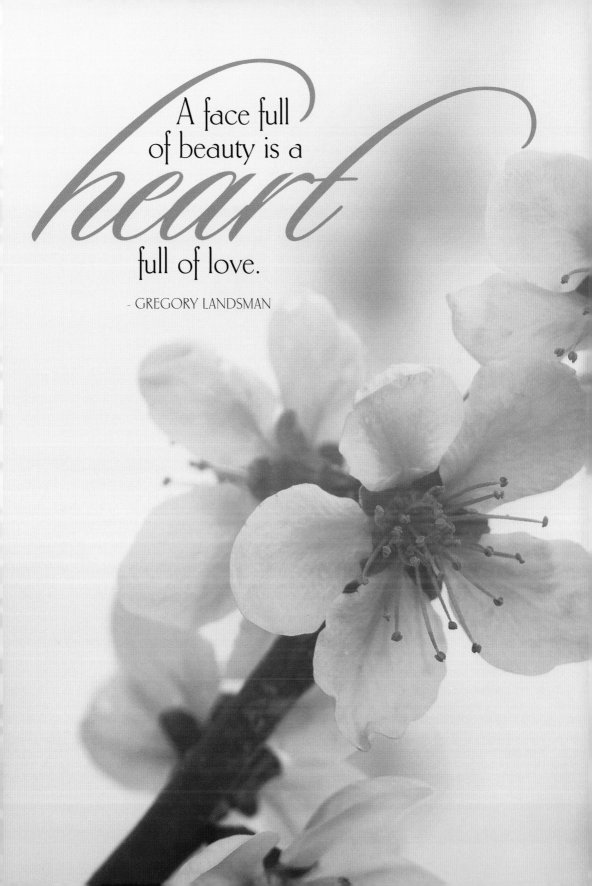

A face full
of beauty is a
heart
full of love.

- GREGORY LANDSMAN

Enthusiasm

Awakening the enthusiastic response within yourself is not about excitement but a deep conviction that what you are and represent is a true reflection of you. The more enthusiasm we feel for ourselves, the more energy we have to participate in life and the more we can express ourselves fully.

Put your heart into everything that you do and remain true to yourself.

- Admire others but never envy them.
- Maintain a sense of humour and practice forgiveness.
- Never argue for your limitations, only your possibilities.
- Believe in your dreams and don't be afraid to follow them even if no one else will.

Acceptance

Acceptance dissolves the limitations and expectations we have on ourselves and others. It is not about reciting affirmations or chanting mantras, it is about making the decision to drop judgment from our lives. Self acceptance is the way we make peace with ourselves.

- Keep good company with yourself and practice sitting in silence for at least 10 minutes every day.
- Think only beauty when you look into a person's eyes, and you will begin to see it when you look into your own.
- Make peace with yourself by giving up self criticism and criticism of others.
- Never be scared to say 'no', as you train people how to treat you by what you allow them to do to you.
- Always stand up for your individuality knowing that the key to your happiness is in holding deep convictions about who you are and what you believe.

Understanding

Understanding ourselves gives us emotional and mental clarity and enables us to honour who we are and the choices we make. Healing our beauty comes first from healing and feeling our beliefs that have stopped us from feeling our beauty.

Through understanding we begin to open up clear channels of communication with ourselves and others, which naturally opens up the way to live authentically.

- Remember that your beauty is not determined by your bone structure but by the structure of your thoughts.
- Concentrate not on how others treat you, but on how you treat yourself.
- Never judge others by their looks, as good looks do not necessarily equate to good people or good love.
- Always choose to be kind – what you give will live in your heart forever.
- Love who you are and all aspects of yourself and don't give that responsibility to anyone else.

Trust

Trust attunes our hearts and minds so that we can strengthen self belief and develop spontaneity, creativity and adventure in our lives.

When you trust in yourself and believe in who you are and love who you are, you begin to affirm trust in the wisdom and love of the God that created you.

- Remember that the most beautiful aspect of a human being can't always be seen with your eyes – your heart is one of them.
- Recognise beauty in the things that you do, not only in the things you have.
- Count your blessings and focus on what you have to give the world, rather than what the world has not given you.
- Remember each day that you are whole and beautiful for no other reason than you are human.

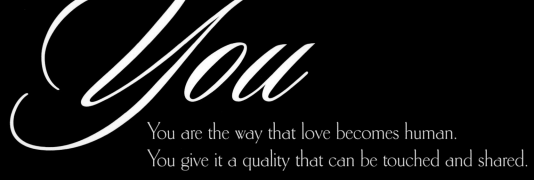

You

You are the way that love becomes human.
You give it a quality that can be touched and shared.

You give love and life meaning.
Use your body to express this love.

Use your heart to feel it, your eyes to see it,
your ears to hear it, your hands to create and share it,
and your feet to be grounded in it.

Take a deep breath, kick off your shoes
and feel the earth under your feet.

Feel the sun and smell the air.

- GREGORY LANDSMAN

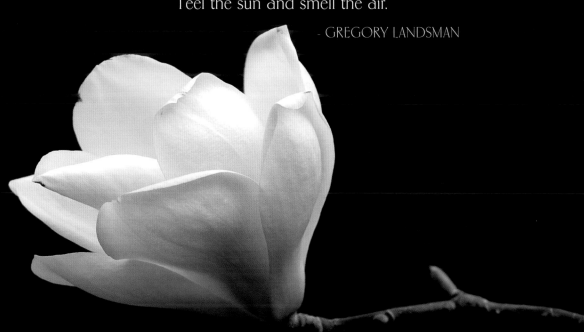

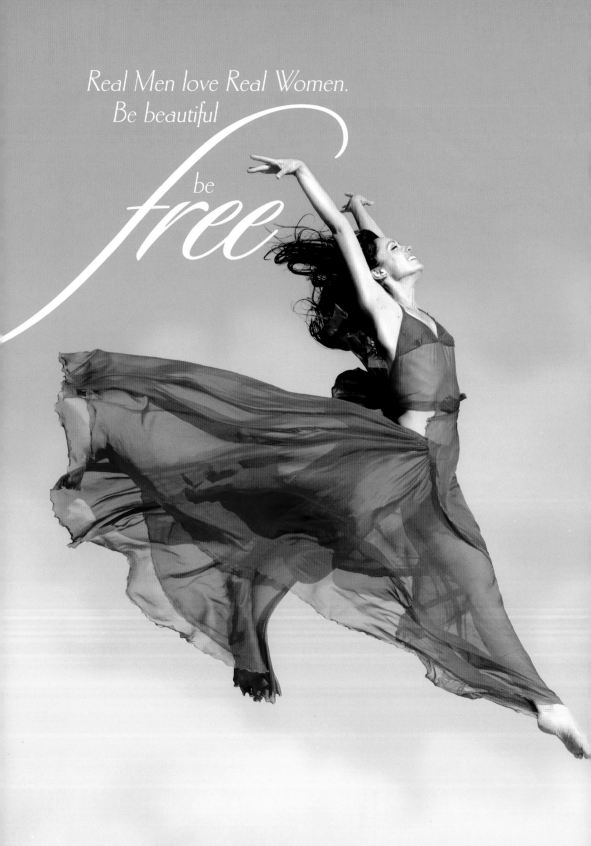

Real Men love Real Women.
Be beautiful

be
free

times

ARE DEFINITELY *changing* AND FOR THE BETTER!

It is becoming increasingly evident that women are no longer feeling the need to conform to the old rigid notions of what makes them beautiful and are no longer judging themselves as harshly.

Just last week I saw a full bodied Goddess step out of the ocean in a bikini. The way she walked let everyone know that the truth of beauty had arrived. It wasn't about her weight, her make up, her hair or her body shape. Her smile, wide and real, was a reminder that the new BEAUTY is about looking the world straight in its face, without making any excuses for who we are or what we look like.

Her partner was waiting on the beach with sun block at the ready and proceeded to rub her back and legs with it. As he moved his hands all over her body, his face had a smile on it like a boy who was eating the best ice cream in the world. There was no doubt that he was loving her up.

It was clear to me (and everyone else on the beach) that this man wasn't looking for any so-called flaws or faults, and her attitude and openness weren't excusing any. He was enjoying her for who she was and she was enjoying herself. Fully present, no excuses, no wishing, no hiding – just beauty expressing itself in its purest form.

Something that many women often forget is that as men we feel very blessed when we have a woman who is willing to share the best of themselves with us. Ask most men and they will tell you that they would trade in an empty relationship with someone whose sole focus is her skinny thighs and waist for a woman who is confident in her own skin with a loving heart.

I believe that the **Real Men** mantra about weight reflects how men often talk to themselves. 'So your belly's not flat, who cares about that, and you're not bone thin, that no sin...'

Upshot – real men love you just the way you are!

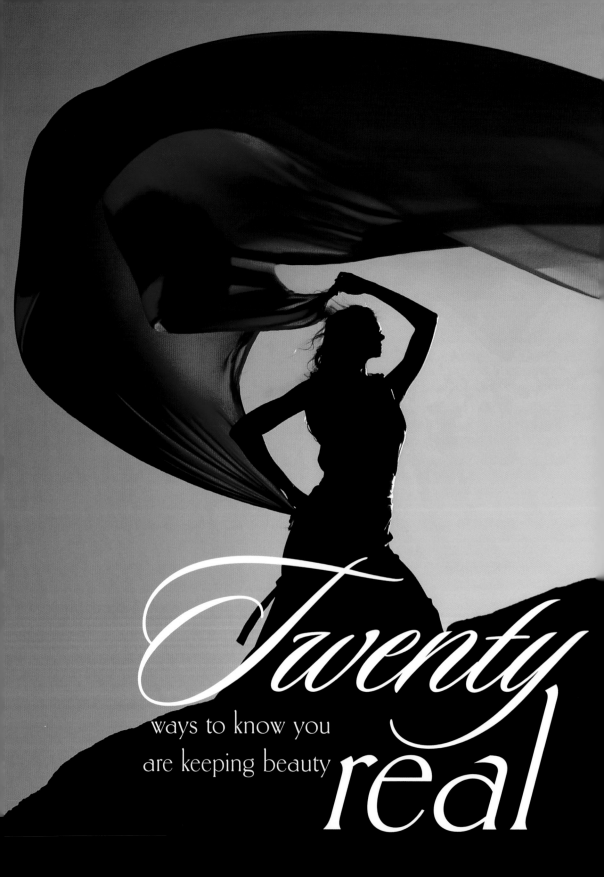

Twenty

ways to know you
are keeping beauty

real

BEAUTY helps us to see how we think, feel, live and love. It has no doctrines; it is a personal journey of liberation and illumination.

One of the greatest challenges in life is to find a way of thinking and living that enables us to reflect, celebrate and express our individuality. I believe this is a journey where we discover aspects of ourselves that we have forgotten.

More often than not we come to think of ourselves as those around us think. These negative thought habits have been learnt. They are not really yours, but have the potential to damage and alter the way you see the world and those around you. But more importantly they can damage how you feel about yourself and make you doubt the essence of what makes you valuable and beautiful. This doubt places limitations on how we express ourselves, see ourselves and live our lives. Living the principles of BEAUTY can help us break down the limitations.

I always believe that awareness is half of the healing as we can then make conscious decisions to move beyond any limitations that we have placed on ourselves.

Our beauty as human beings remains faithful to us when we move towards our individuality and celebrate all that it holds.

1. Balance, Enthusiasm, Acceptance, Understanding, Trust and You urge all of us to celebrate our humanity.
2. BEAUTY demands truth and respect.
3. BEAUTY is life changing when we accept that the most beautiful aspects of who we are cannot always be seen with the eyes.
4. BEAUTY means we choose what we want to buy instead of being manipulated to buy it.
5. BEAUTY means we celebrate who we are and our differences.
6. BEAUTY means addressing real issues without avoiding them.
7. BEAUTY demands that what we pay for gives us results.
8. BEAUTY means accepting that what is in a magazine does not have the power to make us feel bad.
9. BEAUTY means knowing that as human beings we already have beauty.
10. BEAUTY knows that what looks good is not necessarily good for us.
11. BEAUTY knows that we all deserve to be loved for who we are, not what we think others want us to be.
12. BEAUTY gives us the strength and courage to understand our feelings and insecurities and listen to the promise of a new day.
13. BEAUTY knows that we are only as ugly as the judgments we make.
14. BEAUTY is outstanding, outdoing, outlasting the fantasy of beauty every time.
15. BEAUTY knows that there is not a person on Earth that is not touched by beauty.
16. BEAUTY knows we are only as real as the choices we make day-to-day, hour-to-hour, minute-to-minute.
17. BEAUTY knows that we are only beautiful when we look in a mirror and understand that beauty is not tied up with our bone structure but the structure of our thoughts.
18. BEAUTY only has power in life when an individual knows that the beauty they search for outside of themselves is a small aspect of what lies within.
19. BEAUTY knows that as individuals we can make a change, but together we can make a difference.
20. BEAUTY has the power to rapidly transform our inner world and the world we share with others.

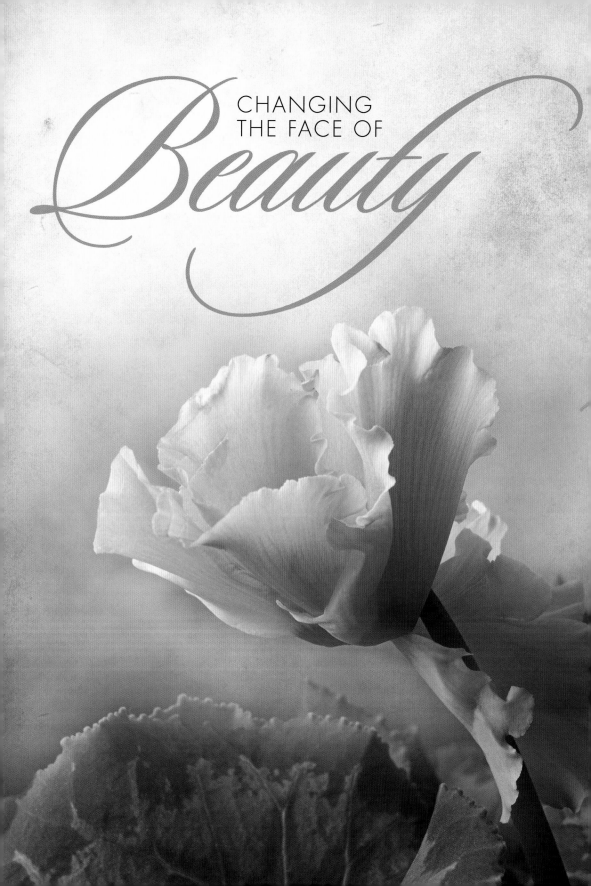

My journey with the concept of beauty has been a long one. It started when I was born into Apartheid ruled South Africa, at a place and time when the colour of your skin determined all that you could hope to be in the world.

Looking back on this journey with many chapters, I can see what drove me from being told that I couldn't get on a certain bus or attend a certain cinema, to working with those heralded for their beauty, to supporting people, and in particular children, to know that their physical body is the smallest aspect of what makes a person truly beautiful.

This is a much longer story, but I wanted to share an important part of my journey that took me to India twenty years ago and started my quest to 'Change the Face of BEAUTY' as we know it.

I had determined to travel to India by myself for a few weeks. It was here in this incredible land of contradictions that I did a great deal of soul searching. In the faces of its people I saw a courageous ability to embrace life, rather than hide from it and to show up for it every day no matter what pain was endured.

I felt an intimate admiration for the strength and courage of these people and their willingness to stand up again and again when life knocked them down. My struggle wasn't theirs, in fact it was nothing like theirs, but still I felt a connectedness in those moments that most people struggle to find their place in the world.

In India, every day is a test of survival, a test of faith. Witnessing poverty and death on the streets made me ask myself question after question in relation to how I had lived my life to date.

If I left the earth today would I believe I had lived a full life?

Had I shared enough of my skills with people?

Is what I did on a day-to-day basis something that contributed to the world being a better place?

I didn't have all the answers, but I handed them over to God, knowing that the answer to those questions would help me to seek the truth about what really makes up a good life.

When I was out taking photographs one day in Madras (as it was then), I noticed a small framed woman standing in the early morning light, untouched and unmoved by all around her, while her sari danced in the wind.

She stood with her back to the sun, glancing over one shoulder, revealing only one side of her face. To me she looked like she had been dropped from heaven wrapped in a rainbow.

There was something oddly familiar about this scene. It reminded me of a fashion shoot where the breeze gently moved the model's garment and she would smile simultaneously, capturing that perfect photographic moment.

But this woman was no model and she certainly wasn't in a glamorous location. She turned, and as if in slow motion, her whole image morphed.

To my dismay I saw that her face had two dramatically different sides that bore no resemblance to each other in any way. The left side was disfigured, showing a mound of purple, saggy flesh that hung over her cheek, forming a drape that concealed any bone structure. Despite this, she turned towards me exuding an air of pride.

Our eyes locked, she smiled at me and then dropped her head to look at a child playing in the mud. With uncertainty in my voice I asked her if she would like her photo taken. Instantly her rich brown face cracked open with a smile that stretched from ear to ear. She nodded, then in a thunderous voice she called out to the entire village. In response almost every man, woman and child gathered around to watch. I focused the camera, and she gently touched her hair to ensure that it was in place.

I admired her eagerness, remembering how I often had to beg friends and relatives to take happy snaps.

Unblinkingly she looked into the lens. Her gaze was so intense it asked me, 'What did this mean?'

I knew what it was to be judged for how you looked, having been beaten and spat on by kids at school in South Africa on a daily basis for the way I looked. Yet in recent years I had lived in a world that placed an exclusive focus on physical beauty; a world where the word 'beauty' was used to justify why some felt privileged and superior, and all because of their fleeting looks.

As I stood there I was witnessing the raw truth of beauty. Staring silently at the sagging muscles on this woman's face I knew I was being challenged by a truth that deep down I had always known, that skin-deep beauty would never be enough.

As I lined up the shot, two tourists stopped and stared with morbid curiosity. Then one said, 'My God isn't nature cruel?' It is so easy to judge what we think is ugly and feel righteous in doing so. In that moment I questioned the nature of cruelty. It was clear that it isn't nature that is cruel, but rather our lack of compassion or acceptance of differences.

Undisturbed the woman smiled for the camera, showing me that I could not change or control someone else's reaction. As she stood with her head high she revealed that she had long ago risen up to meet her beauty and her truth. She was willing to embrace all of who she was and what life had given her, and she was not concerned about how others responded.

As I took her photograph I studied her face. Her appearance disturbed me as it brushed up against everything we are taught about what makes someone valuable. But when I looked into her eyes I felt deeply moved. She had a sense of calm acceptance and integrity that I had never seen on any model's face I had ever worked on, mine included. This woman was living in a cushion of self acceptance; a living example that the essence of our beauty lies not in our physical characteristics, but in the heart of our character.

Looking at her I was filled with a longing for something that I did not yet truly know and wondered how liberating it must be to have such a sense of peace within one's self; to leave behind the impossible ideals of physical perfection that so often stops us feeling good about ourselves. I could see so clearly the reality of beauty and in that moment a part of me vowed to help others do the same.

This woman held up beauty, hope, acceptance and courage amidst chaos, confusion, poverty and judgment. I saw what we are all taught is to forget that beauty can shine through every face, because the power and the true essence of beauty unfolds from the inside out.

When I had finished taking the photos, this wondrous woman placed both her hands together in the middle of her chest, lowered her head slightly, smiled and walked away.

I sat on the sidewalk after and wrote what this teacher of true beauty had taught me:

In life sometimes love presents itself in a form that is totally unexpected.

Rise to the consciousness of the love, not the level of the form.

Whenever I am tempted to judge someone I remind myself of this.

The day I left Puttaparthi, this wonderful teacher of beauty was there to farewell me. She waved to the man who had reminded the village that she was valuable enough to be photographed, and I waved goodbye to the woman who taught me the power of gratitude.

Still today when I give too much thought to the way I look, I close my eyes and remember a woman who was proud and victorious in who she was and what she represented in the world, and I affirm silently that a face full of beauty is a heart full of love.

In remembering this we are all free.

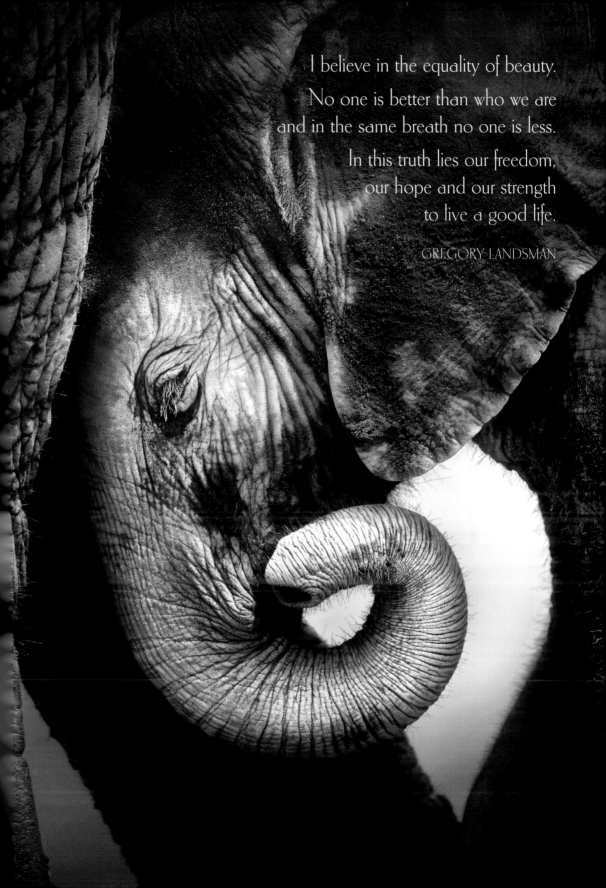

I believe in the equality of beauty.
No one is better than who we are
and in the same breath no one is less.

In this truth lies our freedom,
our hope and our strength
to live a good life.

GREGORY LANDSMAN

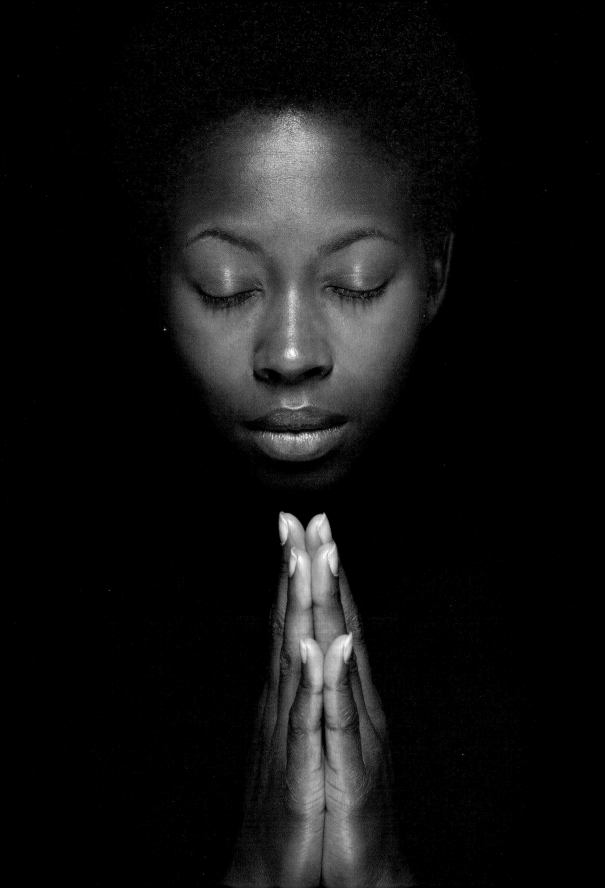

Love and beauty are interlinked,
with one you ultimately share the other.

You are the way that beauty becomes human.

You give it a quality that can be touched and shared.

You give love and beauty meaning.

Use your body to

express

this beauty.

Use your heart to feel it,
your eyes to see it,
your ears to hear it,
your hands to create and share it,
and your feet to be grounded in it.

– GREGORY LANDSMAN

HOW TO RELIEVE
stress
IN 5 MINUTES

Most of us have our own ways of dealing with stress and that often involves hitting the gym, a punching bag or the treadmill for an hour. But if you haven't got the time and you are feeling stressed, try the following 5 minute de-stress and age-less solutions.

Hug someone you love

This is a simple but powerful stress reliever because it brings on the release of the happy hormone oxytocin, which increases trust, acceptance and compassion and in the process relieves stress. Not bad for something that costs nothing and gives so much, not only to you but the person you are hugging! So what are you waiting for, everyone needs a hug!

Breathe in calm

At the end of a stressful day we can feel overloaded and any negative thoughts or emotions that came with the day can create tension and anxiety. Whatever the emotion, feel it, heal it and then let the anger go. If you don't have time for a long deep breathing session do my 5-8-9 technique. Sit down. Keep your back straight, breathe in for a count of 5, hold your breath for a count of 8, and then exhale for 9. Repeat this for a couple of minutes. Making your exhale a few counts longer than your inhale calms your nervous system.

Animal kindness

Our four legged friends (dogs and cats) raise our serotonin and dopamine levels that have calming properties. Loving these little friends reduces depression and calms us down while lowering our blood pressure. Thank heavens they don't charge us for all the goodness they bring to our lives!

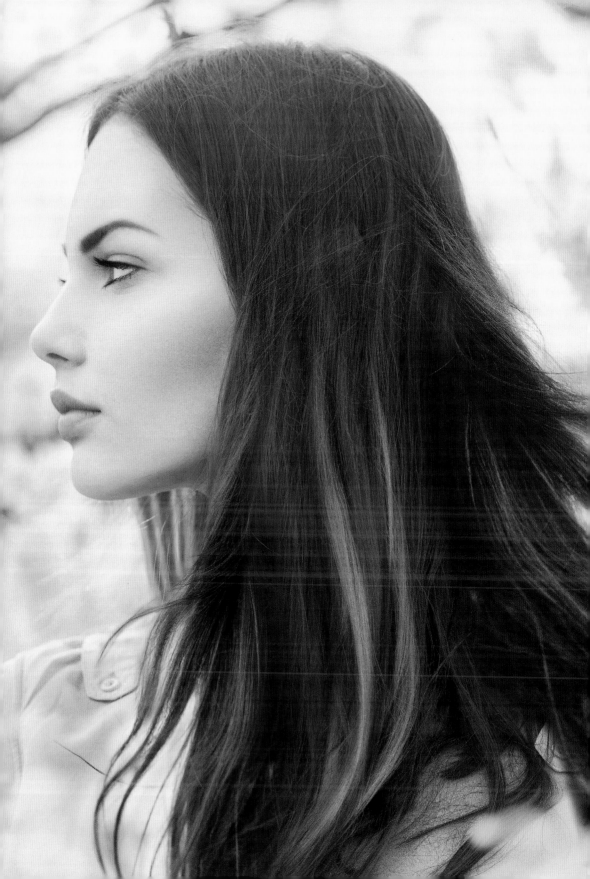

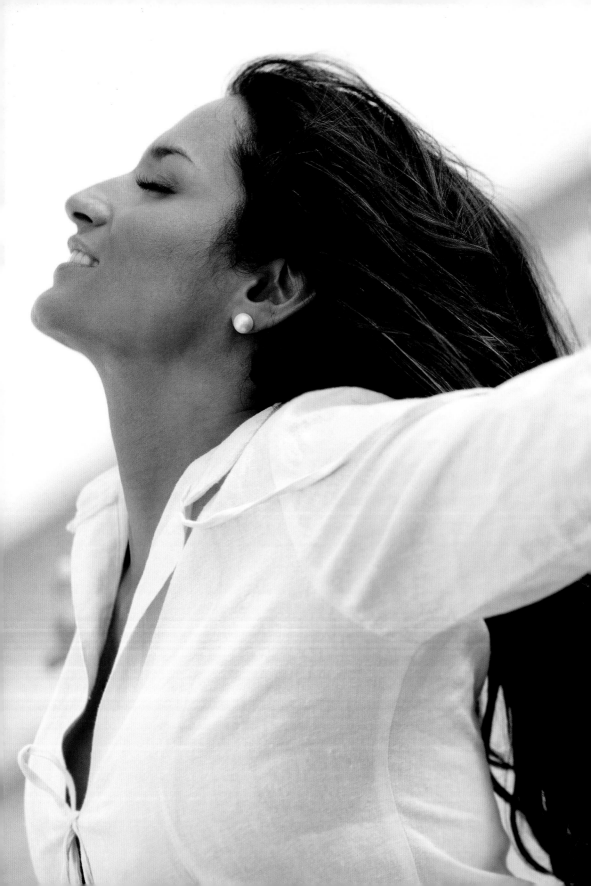

SPREAD YOUR BEAUTY

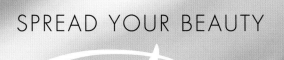

Wings

AND FLY

I met a woman recently who had a deep interest in butterflies. She went on to explain the basics to me. They start off as caterpillars, eating their way through leaves then cocoon themselves and eventually turn into butterflies.

What I didn't know was that to turn from a caterpillar into a butterfly is a feat of nature, a process that takes an extraordinary struggle for the butterfly to break out of the cocoon. But that struggle has a purpose. It strengthens the butterfly's wings so that when it finally breaks free from the cocoon, it is able to fly. She explained to me that if nature had created an easier process for the butterfly its wings would never be strong enough and it would die.

Much like the butterfly, strengthening our own beauty wings is a personal journey that with all its challenges takes us closer to the truth of what makes us beautiful human beings. This can be challenging and often we look at situations and wonder why do things have to be so difficult? Why are so many of us challenged in this area of our lives, never feeling as though we look how we would like to?

My own path through the world has shown me that for most of us there is a certain amount of struggle before we reach a point where we are strong enough to simply be free and fly as God intended us.

So on those days when you are feeling challenged, for something simple or more significant, try to keep in mind that you are strengthening your beauty wings and getting ready to fly.

Be BEAUTIFUL, Be Free…

Don't question your beauty or tear it apart.
It serves you no purpose,
Except to pull at your heart.
Beauty is simple just look at the sun,
Look at the children,
You'll see it is meant to be fun.
It's about laughing and feelings inside.
It's taking those feelings and expressing them outside.
So think about your beauty before you pull it apart,
It serves no purpose,
Except to pull at your heart.
Stop for a minute and listen to your heart.
For it is trying to tell you,
This is where your beauty can start.
Look in the mirror, don't reject what you see.

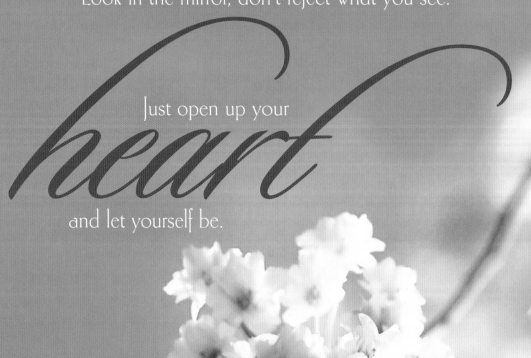

Just open up your

heart

and let yourself be.

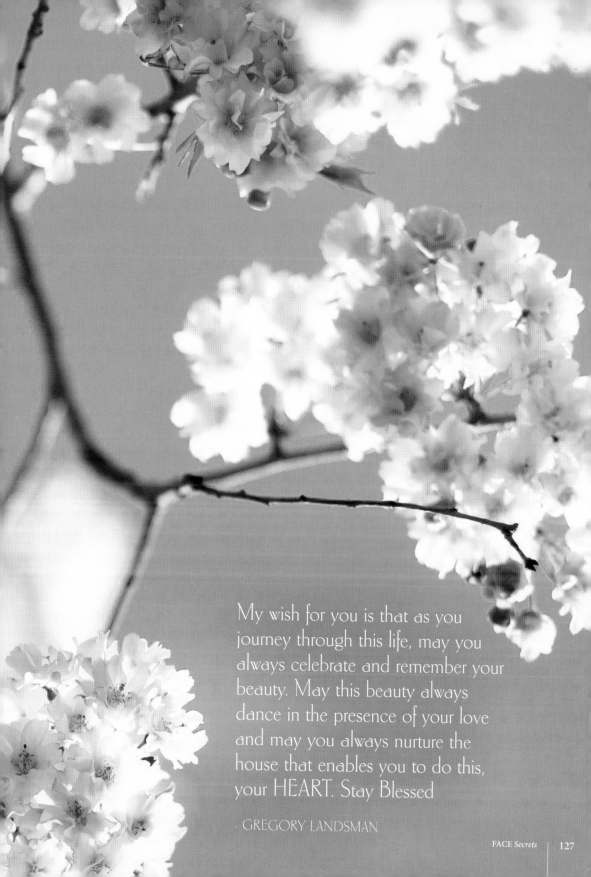

My wish for you is that as you journey through this life, may you always celebrate and remember your beauty. May this beauty always dance in the presence of your love and may you always nurture the house that enables you to do this, your HEART. Stay Blessed

- GREGORY LANDSMAN

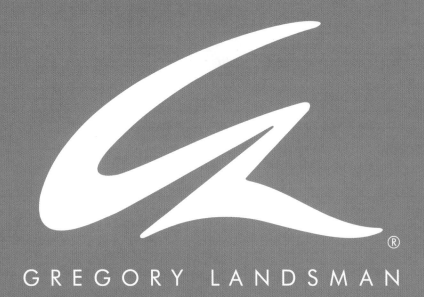

GREGORY LANDSMAN

The GL SKINFIT INSTITUTE® works towards helping
everyone regardless of their age to look younger,
feel younger and stay younger, inside and out.

To read about the 5 Day Face Firming Formula
used by models internationally go to:
www.glskinfitinstitute.com